Amazing Truth About Us

by

Lynne Blighton B.Soc.Wk., Grad. Cert ASWP, AMHSW

Illustrated by Philip Farley

Published by Lynne Blighton

Information contained in this book is covered by trademarks: The Fragile Puzzle™

When families are happy – their radiance reflects into society™

Dedicated to all who value peace and freedom and to my late cousin Judy (on my mother's side) who encouraged me to write this book in a simplistic form. Judy passed before seeing the final production.

Amazing Truth About Us
Hardback Edition June 2018
ISBN 978-0-9585965-9-6
Mobi ISBN 978-0-6482994-0-0
EPUB ISBN 978-0-6482994-2-4

Published by Lynne Blighton
PO Box 725, Cleveland, Qld 4163 Australia
© 2018 Lynne Blighton B Soc Wk, Grad Cert ASWP, AMHSW

Acknowledgments
My gratitude and thanks to my editor Jean Wilson and to my early content reader Michele Hart. Their talent has put sparkle into this book. I would like to acknowledge the important part played by my cousin the late Judy Bonnett who passed away in 2017. Judy inspired me in 2016 to write in 'children's story book' style. She said I was to keep it short and simple, so the world could understand what I was talking about. I cannot say enough about how hard it was to write such a complex subject in a few pages of text, but I think it worked. Thank you to Philip Farley whose colourful illustrations tell a story of our Earth's journey and human influence. Thank you to David Rosenorn and Adam Livings for their professional approach and eye for detail which filled me with confidence. Thank you both for making a scary process into a fun adventure. Thank you to my friends who encouraged me keep going on those days when it all seemed so pointless. Book writing can be a thankless task, hours and hours on your own while your friends have a life. Never mind, my turn is coming soon!

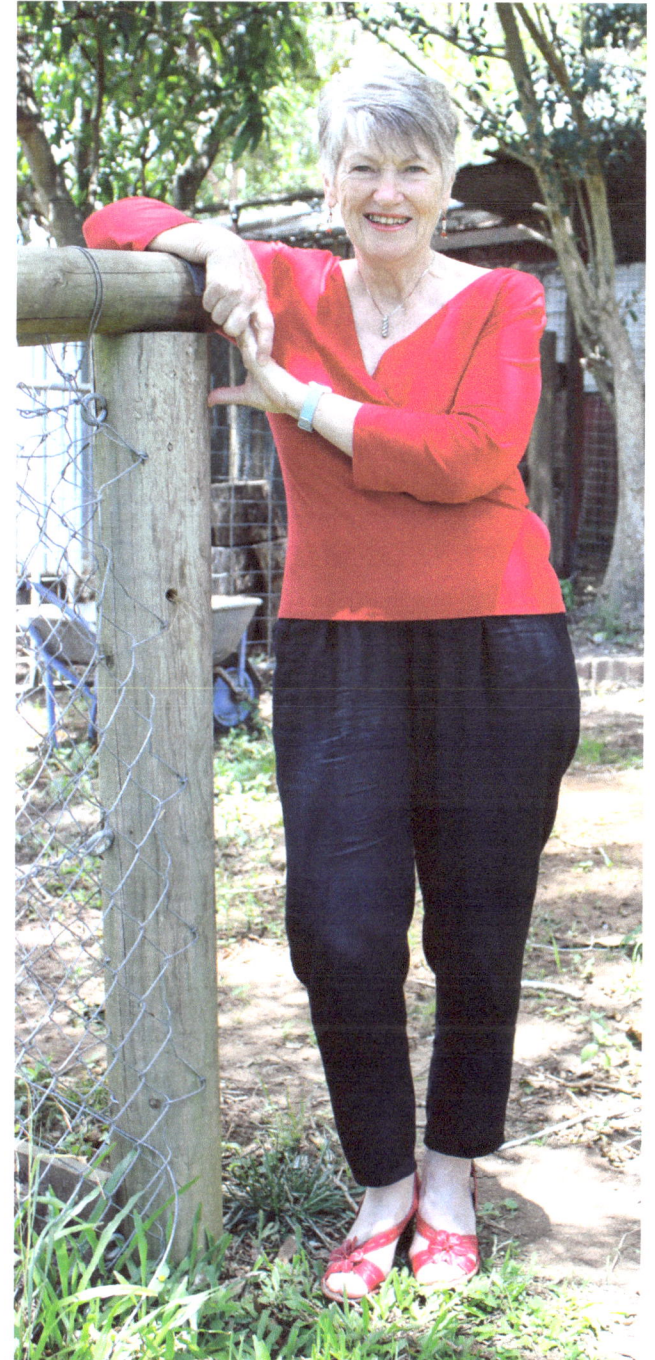

THE AUTHOR

Lynne Blighton was conceived during World War II and born after the war ended. She was often parked outside shops in her pram alongside wheelchair bound returned soldiers with body parts missing or violently shaking with shell shock. There was an agreement in the village to not hide their wounded behind closed doors, but those awful sights strongly impacted her young mind. Lynne remained in Tiptree, Essex, England until her early twenties when she set off on an adventure around the world, leaving with one question on her mind: Why are people like they are?

Lynne settled in Australia living in Brisbane, Queensland. At age 35 Lynne was accepted into the University of Queensland to study Social Work focusing her study on Group and Family Therapy. After graduating Lynne opened her own therapy centre and developed a method of communicating complex theories through simplistic drawings. She continued her studies to gain a Graduate Certificate in Advanced Social Work Practice, later becoming an Accredited Mental Health Social Worker with eligibility to take medical practitioner referrals. In 1997 Lynne returned to her beloved England and worked as a social worker in London for five years until she needed to look after her elderly mother in Western Australia; returning to Queensland after her mother's death. 'My house had been a rental for many years and was left in such a mess.' After securing a part-time job with the Queensland Government Lynne started renovating and continued to see clients and develop The Fragile Puzzle™ books and product range in her private time.

In 2014 Lynne learned that human beings are symbiotic organisms created from two entirely different organisms living as one organism for survival. This knowledge opened a new world of understanding of the method she had created. Today Lynne is on a new pathway transforming her work into a language that talks about body cells and bacterial cells. Amazingly this knowledge has always been at the base of The Fragile Puzzle™ which teaches people to distinguish between two entirely different forms of communication that happen simultaneously within our body. Lynne has dedicated her lifetime to discovering the secrets of life which she shares through her work which is captured in The Fragile Puzzle™ books, products, webinars and podcasts. People around Lynne often comment about her abundant supply of energy and amazing vitality and wonder how she has managed to keep up her enthusiasm along such a long journey. This book is a step in a new direction for Lynne's work, into the world of bacteria.

The format of a story book for adults provides a base to articulate extremely complex information in a semi-factual style. It gives you Lynne's knowledge of why people are like they are.

Lynne B

THE ILLUSTRATOR

Born in Brisbane in 1960, Philip's artistic talent was soon recognised and he was given private tuition in creative art. After three years at the Queensland College of Art, Philip initially became an illustrator. For the last 30 years he has been a full time fine artist. His skills and the emotional impact of his work have led to over a dozen state and national art awards and growing public appreciation.

"Whether it's a landscape, portrait, wildlife or city scape, I try to capture the effects of light and colour to convey the essence and character of the subject matter. This can be created by fine detail and the use of accuracy, other times through broader brush strokes/bold colours."

Philip Farley

art@philipfarley.com
www.philipfarley.com

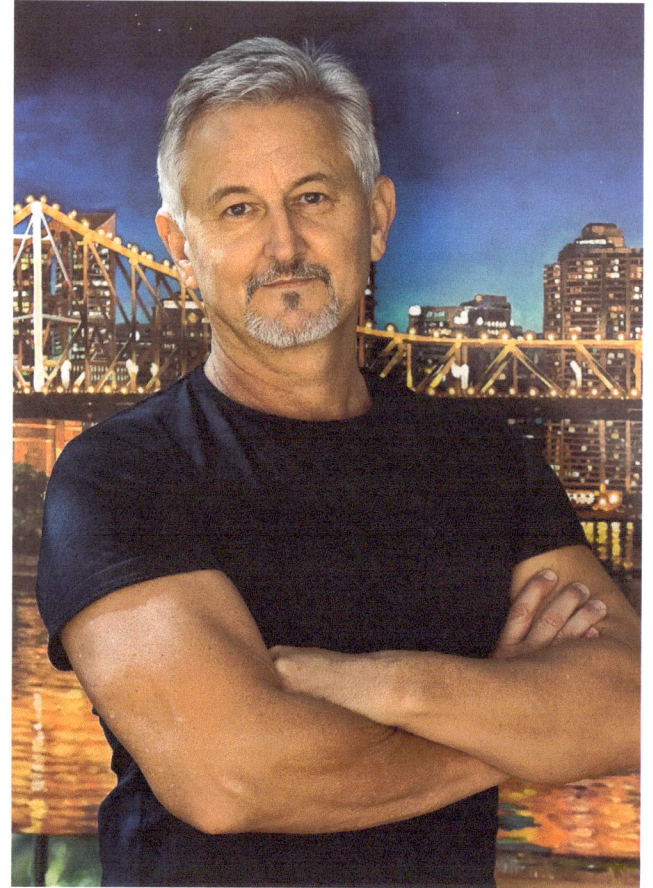

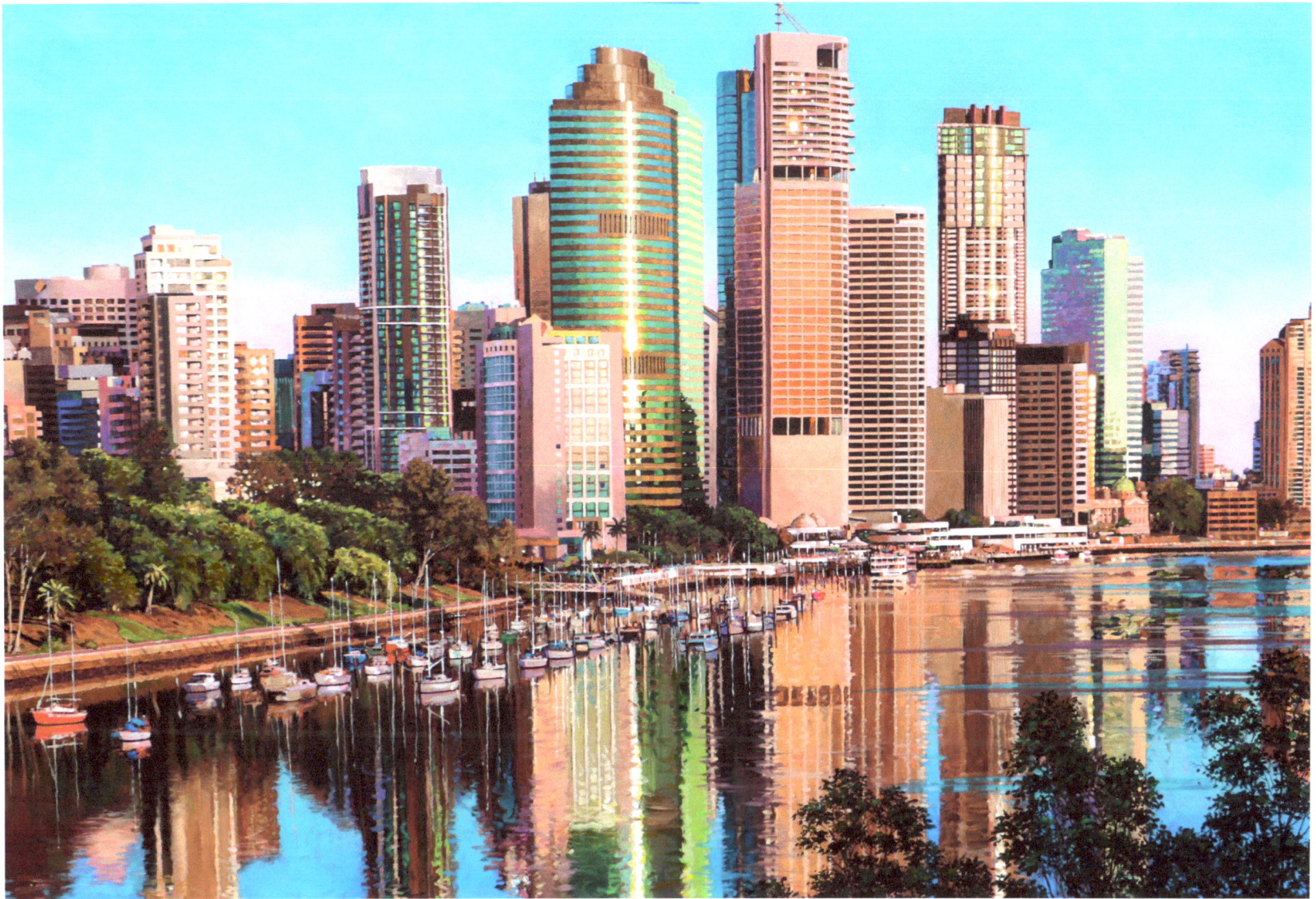

Brisbane Morning

by Philip Farley

Contents

Story Preparation – A Message from Lynne

At its heart, my work assists clients to become aware of the existence of a survival mechanism which has links to pre-historic knowledge stored in our DNA. This part is so strong within us that should it sense the need to keep us safe, it automatically instantly over-rides all current thoughts and feelings as it clicks us into fight or flight mode to prepare us to run like hell or stand and fight off attackers. Although our survival mechanism is part of us it doesn't feel quite the same within our system as our other parts. I cannot describe this 'difference' in words but can sense it in myself and others.

I guide clients to identify the 'difference' by showing them how to recognise when and why their survival mechanism has been activated. What often happens is the person's own fears activate their survival mechanism putting them in a loop to nowhere. I encourage clients to welcome their survival mechanism and thank it for looking after them 24/7; learn to trust it and discover how it uses subtle messages through the gut to guide us to the truth. I caution my clients to give up all ideas of fighting this part. NEVER try to control it – they quickly learn the consequences of not following this sound advice. After a few struggles with ego, most clients acquire great respect for the ability this part has to flip their life into a spin unexpectedly. I teach clients to recognise when they have accidentally triggered fight or flight; and how to stop triggering false alarms. Gradually clients realise most of their emotional problems were caused by self-created false alarms.

A cathartic moment happens when confusion melts away and is replaced with an amazing new sense of self confidence, self-assuredness, inner harmony and emotional balance. The work usually leaves clients glowing with health and well-being, all achieved by learning what parts of the self to control and what not to control. It all starts with recognition of the different feelings and emotions within us; knowing what feelings to listen to and what not to listen to – and learning how to maintain balance between the two.

Although achieving brilliant results I could not articulate what I was doing other than teaching people to communicate with their survival mechanism. I knew the why, but not the what. In July 2014 a massive realisation left me stunned. Did you know that human beings are symbiotic organisms made from two entirely different organisms that live as one? We are formed from bacteria and human cells – which was hard to get my head around but made perfect sense of why there are two entirely different communication sensations within our body. Suddenly I understood why 'balance' between the two sides has always been so important for our physical and mental health and wellbeing.

I sense that when people can find and maintain emotionally well-balanced responses to life, this changes their gut flora which improves the health of the entire system. To share my knowledge with the world I have chosen to write a very short easily understood book in the form of a play with fictitious characters that can articulate extremely complex information in a semi factual style. What follows has absolutely nothing to do with how I work with clients but does mirror the knowledge base that guides my work. Hopefully my short story will assist you in understanding the fragility of your own internal communication systems and the effect these ultimately have on our society. Hopefully my work will reframe how we view 'bacteria' which is a massive part of who we are.

My story aims to leave readers with a clear understanding of 'what does what' within our system so that readers can gain a clear sense of what to take control of, and what must NEVER be controlled. Getting these basics right has been the corner stone of success for my clients to move them from emotional chaos to emotional harmony.

Lynne B

Scene One – Building Our Foundation

Are you sitting comfortably as we go down a strange pathway to unfold a story about you, me and every other human being on our planet. The story takes us back to the beginning of life on earth and is the story of two microscopic organisms, bacteria and soft floppy single cell creatures that joined forces millions of years ago and eventually evolved into human beings. The soft floppy ones didn't have much shape unlike the stronger more fibrous bacteria – however both were highly intelligent, and both used electricity to communicate with others of their kind.

Bacteria developed many different shapes and forms and covered every nook and cranny on the Earth. Some developed into kind bacteria and others became ruthless highly efficient killers that destroyed everything in their path, including the kind bacteria and single cell soft floppy creatures. The killer bacteria knew a lot about chemistry and manufactured deadly excretions to make other life forms deteriorate and rot; a perfect place to grow more bacteria. It was a very scary place to live.

Then one eventful day, probably quite by accident, a kind bacteria met up with a soft floppy single cell creature and both were immediately attracted to each other. In fact, they literally became absorbed by each other. When their slightly different electrical currents met, this caused a great electrical spark of magnificent light which radiated throughout both organisms and beyond. It was a powerful living electrical energy which bonded them together.

We know this living energy as our spirit and the explosion of energy released feelings of LOVE and sexual energy; it was probably the world's first love story. Of course, living in such a dangerous world, both organisms already knew a lot about FEAR which triggered the need to hide. Both organisms were entranced by their new vibrations. Sexual energy released vitality and LOVE made them feel safe and strong, creating a powerful bond that fused the kind bacteria and the soft floppy cells into a beautiful living energy mass.

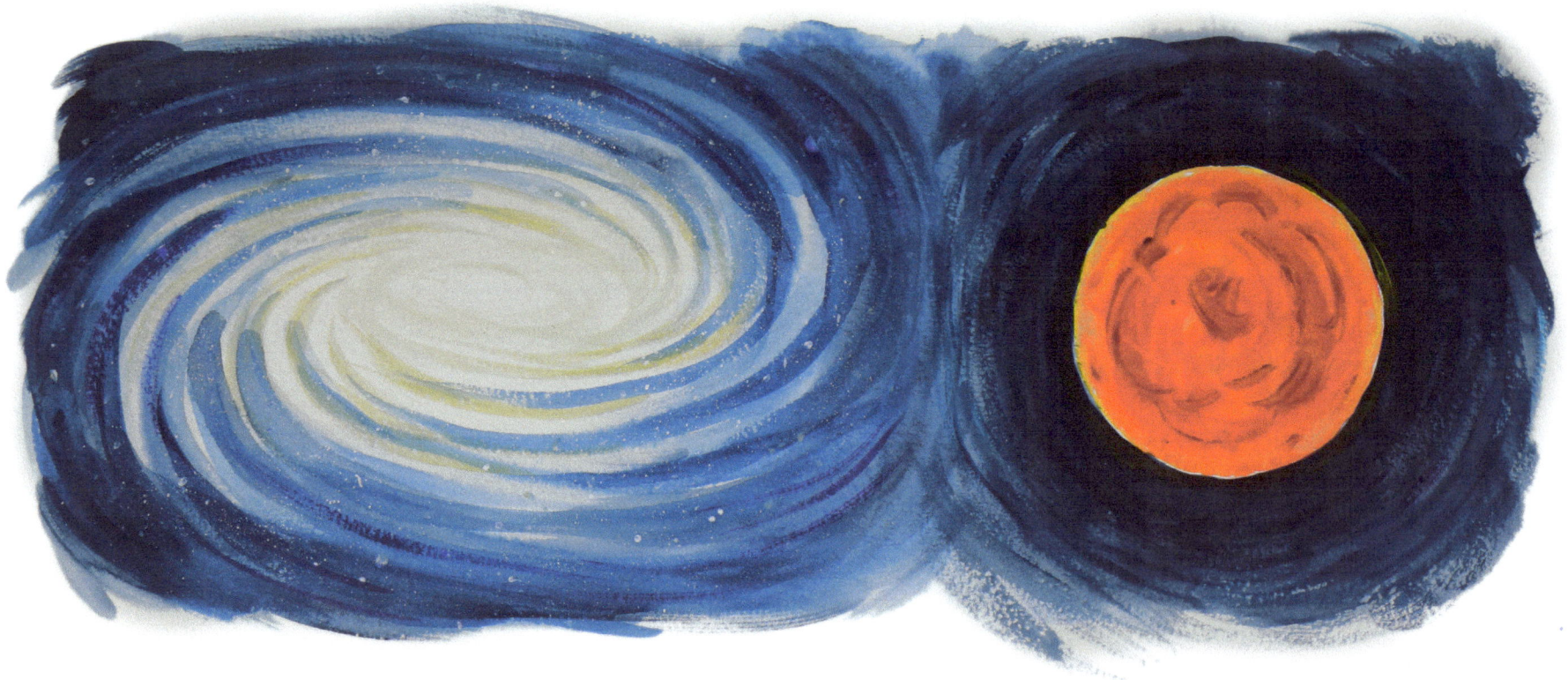

It was perfect for procreation and the combined organisms (known as a symbiotic organism) grew quickly. The kind bacteria grew slightly faster and soon surrounded the soft floppy cells to protect them from killer bacteria; and soon they outnumbered soft floppy cells at the ratio of 10:1. The soft floppy cells didn't mind because the kind bacteria formed an army to protect them. The kind bacteria were so brave and greatly admired by the soft floppy cells. As the symbiotic organism continued to grow it developed incredible new structures by sharing different attributes and special knowledge. They formed skin around the body mass to keep all the cells together. The skin was cleverly designed to let food and oxygen in but keep killer bacteria out and could even excrete waste and excess water to wash itself clean. A marvelous advancement for life on Earth!

Each organism had different ways of communicating:

- The kind bacteria were highly telepathic and used electrical currents to transmit and receive messages through the airwaves – a bit like radio, mobile phones and television. They picked up vibes from the wider world to maintain a strong sense of what was going on around them which was a huge bonus for the symbiotic organism. It could also be used to communicate with others of their kind and pre-empt dangerous situations.

- The soft floppy cells communicated internally by firing off negatively and positively charged chemicals to create waves of energy which caused vibrations within their fluid filled soft floppy cells. Vibrations in one cell could set off vibrations in neighbouring cells to pass information to the mass of cells. The vibration could even manage a little bodily movement towards or away from things. A very useful skill but limited in application.

Their favourite vibrations were the feelings of LOVE that bound the two together and enabled them to communicate with each other. As the organisms grew the kind bacteria used their slightly more fibrous structure to form electrical pathways (our nervous system) so that electrical currents could be used to safely direct messages to and from various parts of the body. The messages were carried in vibrations experienced by the soft floppy cells, and recorded by the kind bacteria, then stored as memories of past events. Some memories were filled with LOVE and some were filled with FEAR, but these were only 'memories' and not the real thing.

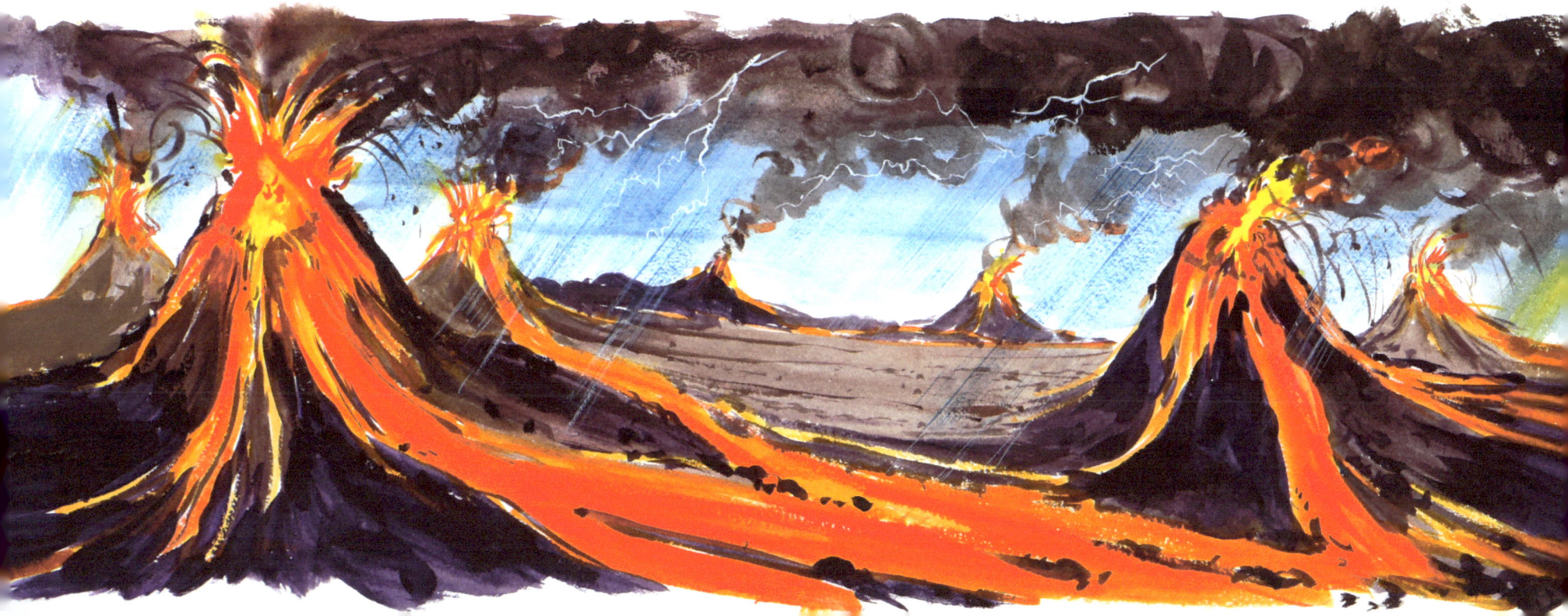

The memories were stored in a 'data storage centre' which we call the brain. The FEAR filled memories could be used to protect the organism. For example, if the highly telepathic kind bacteria sensed approaching danger they could recall and replay a memory of a fearful event to motivate the organism to move away before the danger was upon them. It was such a clever idea and worked well for millions of years. So, in a nutshell, the kind bacteria found ways to use feelings and emotions stored in memories to trigger responses in the body. This was achieved by 'replaying' the vibration stored in the memory throughout the body of cells to recreate the emotional sensation of FEAR ahead of when that sensation would be normally have been felt – sort of like a mock FEAR to trigger a response to danger before the danger was upon them. What a terrific value add!

The kind bacteria and soft floppy cells worked as a team using this wonderfully uncomplicated system built on FEAR and LOVE; fear activated the organisms to move away from danger and LOVE put the organism into a fabulously relaxed state. Full relaxation released sexual energy which pulsed throughout both organisms bringing a wonderful sensation of life and vitality. The symbiotic organism adored this sensation and they grew quickly developing new parts all the time. The biggest looming problem was how to feed the rapidly growing mass – especially those cells in the middle and getting rid of waste was becoming a nightmare! The combined intelligence of the organism found a brilliant solution by forming a long tube right through the centre of the body mass – a bit like a stretched-out hole longways through a sausage.

The kind bacteria found clever ways not to be eaten by killer bacteria and guarded the inner surfaces of the tube. The kind bacteria became very efficient at using pre-recorded vibrations (memory emotions) to guide the body mass towards food which always had killer bacteria all over it. Both food and killer bacteria went into the tube. This brilliant plan utilised the killer bacteria to break down the food into microscopic pieces which the kind bacteria were able to pass through special openings in the tube wall. They used the same system in reverse to pass waste materials into the tube. The killer bacteria continued to break the waste down before everything in the tube was passed out the other end and became compost to help newly forming plants to grow. We call this tube our 'intestines' which starts at our mouth and ends at our bottom. What a terrific system; such mastery over a hostile environment. No wonder this new life form continued to flourish.

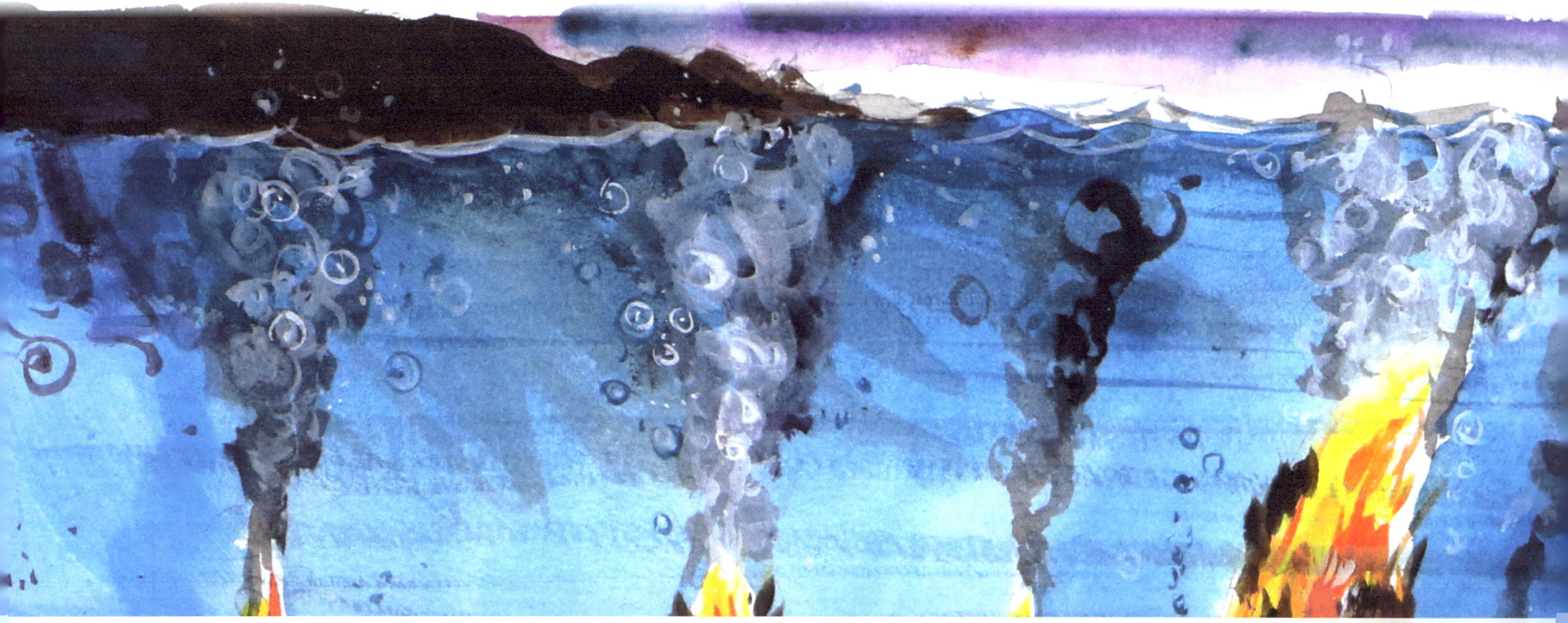

The partnership developed all manner of things: soon the body had developed blood vessels to transport food, oxygen and water all around the body, a pump to keep it all moving, ears to hear the world outside and a nose to smell it. The kind bacteria created an immune system that could wrap invading killer bacteria in mucus to make them harmless until they could be passed out with the waste. The kind bacteria would do anything to protect their beloved body of soft floppy cells which provided them with a comfortable, warm and safe mobile home. The combined organisms even found ways to put thousands of nerve endings into eyes that could take pictures of the outside world. Each picture was stored with full memory of the emotions, smells, sounds, even the temperature at the time the picture was taken. The photos delivered a complex mixture of information which was a great advancement for the kind bacteria who only needed to flash a picture with a particular emotional memory to trigger a rapid response which vibrated throughout the entire body mass. The same system, combined with telepathy, was used to inform the body mass of what was happening in the outside world. It was a huge improvement and so necessary for continued survival in this dangerous environment.

What the organism most needed was the ability to move quickly. They pooled their knowledge to create hard bony structures and found ways to form muscle strands which they strapped to the bones with sinews; putting joints in the bones provided flexibility. It was amazing, but best of all, by implanting nerves with receptors in one end, located in the brain, and receptors in the other end located in the muscles, the kind bacteria were able to use their electrical currents to create movement. Information stored in the memory could be used to send electrical messages through the nerves to trigger the muscles to make them contract and relax the muscle bundles which created movement – the first of its kind on Earth!

The kind bacteria placed receptors all over the body – particularly in the skin so that information from the outside world could be received 24/7 and sent directly to the data storage area (the brain). It was amazing – like wiring a house for the first time. The kind bacteria even used their slightly more fibrous structure to form antennae on the outside of the mass to pick up vibrations from the world. We call these hairs.

A special boney jointed tube (our backbone) was used to protect the main part of the nervous system which was becoming quite complex. The newly emerging

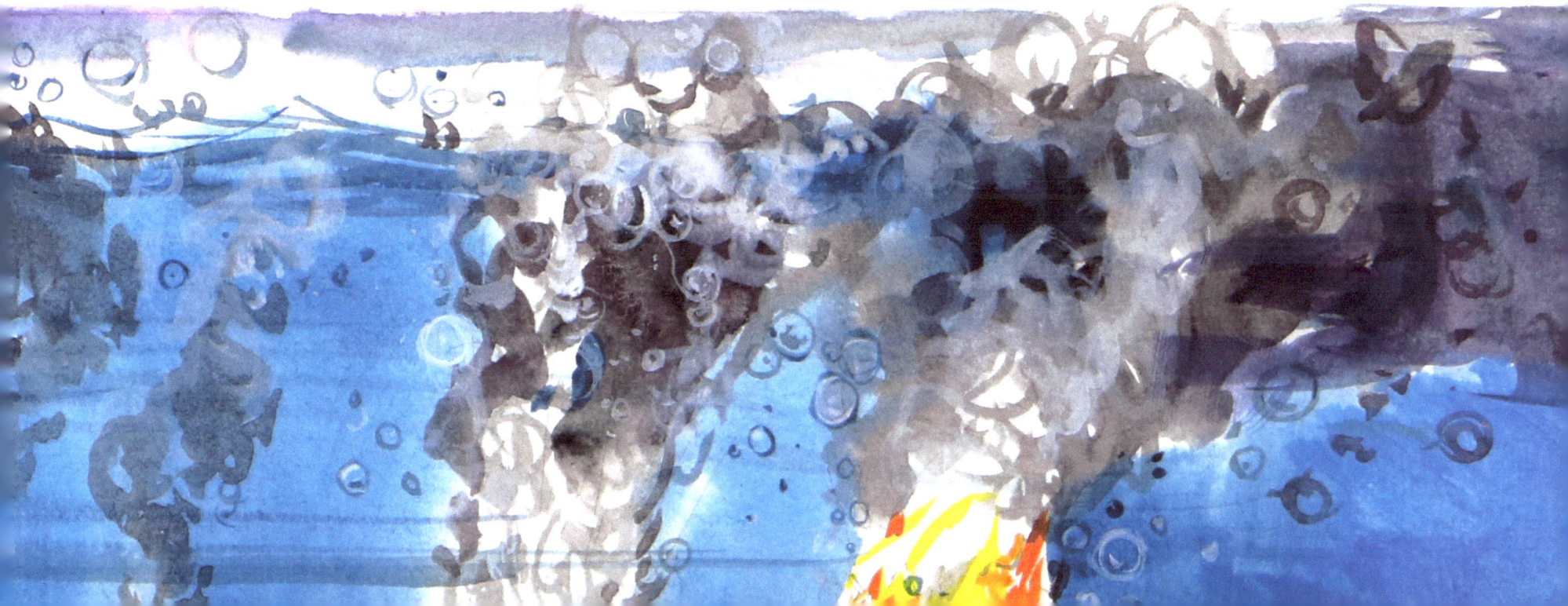

creature was able to raise its body from the ground and run. Freedom to move at last! The symbiotic organism, now in the form of an early mammal roamed the earth and found plenty of food and water which it converted into compost to form a rich layer of soil over the bare rocks so that plants could grow abundantly to create more food to eat. As mammals evolved they developed into various shapes and sizes to adapt to their surroundings; some became animals while others became fish, birds, reptiles and amphibians – the common feature being a backbone and spinal cord. The animals developed teeth to tear and grind food into small parts which were pounded by a massive tongue muscle to mix in special chemicals to start the digestive process. The intestine became very sophisticated and home to all manner of bacteria (some killer and some kind) which we call our gut flora which breaks down food in our internal food processing factory. The kind bacteria created all sorts of appetites which were held in the memory to drive the animals to food and shelter – even organised taste buds on the tongue with neurological links directly to memories of what had been eaten before. A message could be sent at the speed of light – spit that out, it's not safe to eat and will give you a belly ache!

There was so much development happening, but from the beginning of time it was recorded in specialist storage areas which we call DNA. Each organism had their own DNA however the kind bacteria had 10 times more DNA than soft floppy body cells which is probably why the kind bacteria had more control over the symbiotic organism. Their control included using emotions to build habitual behaviour patterns into memory. Habitual behaviour patterns made it easier to manage and organise each species into safe daily routines. These routines could be passed from generation to generation to keep them alive in a hostile world. Survival relied on their ability to accurately predict situations and respond by fighting opponents or running away quickly.

The kind bacteria developed a special early warning system based on the emotion of FEAR. When the system was triggered by FEAR special chemicals were released into the body to close down function in some areas and increase function in others. We call this the Para-sympathic Nervous System, PNS for short and more commonly known as the fight or flight response. It immediately closes down the gut while increasing function in the lungs, kidneys, liver and heart to provide the body with lots of sugar and oxygen to burn as energy to fight or run away fast from danger.

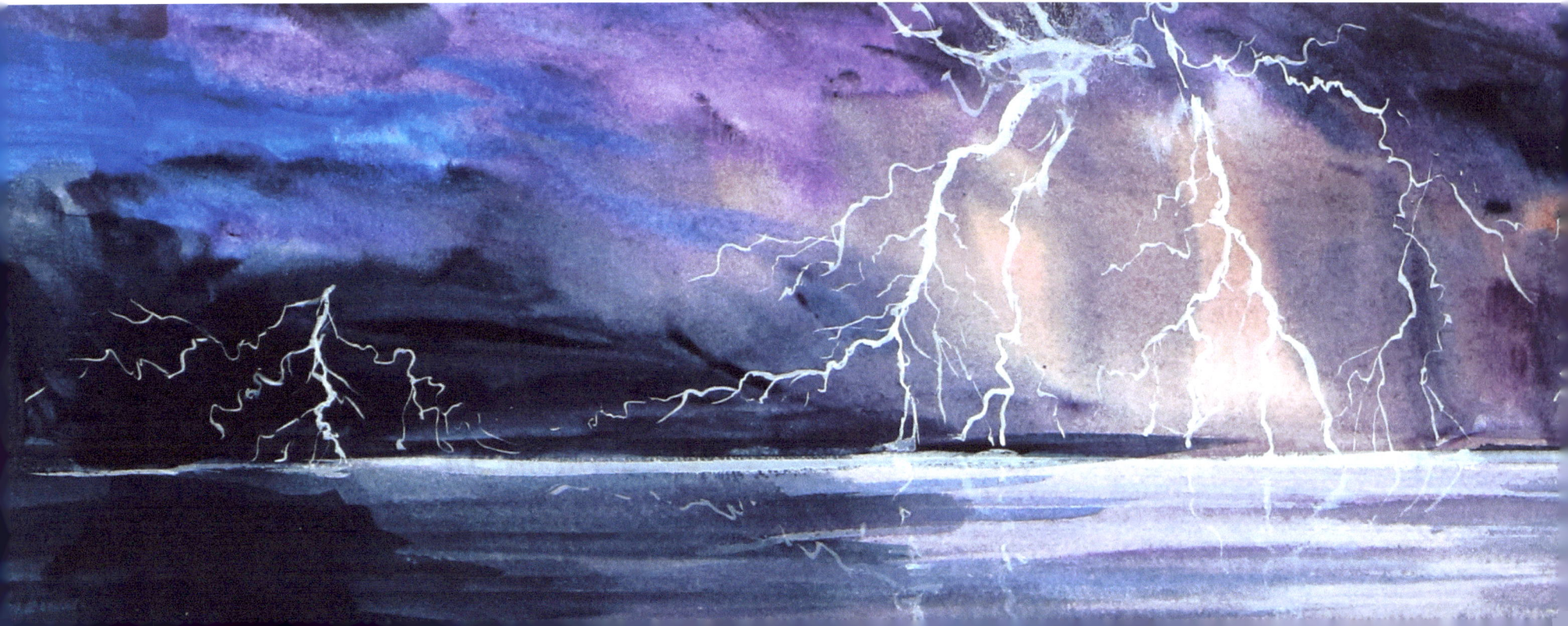

The kind bacteria could easily trigger a fight or flight response by taking a memory from the brain containing feelings and emotions of FEAR. The memory released a flood of fearful feelings and emotions into the body of cells to activate movement. This highly successful response kept the organism alive and evolving for millions more years. Fight and flight is the basic instinct of all mammal related species, including us. Although the animals, birds, fish, reptiles and amphibians occasionally fought aggressively to survive or secure a mate (and sometimes different species ate each other) all were filled with feelings of LOVE which released sexual energy and kept them emotionally and physically well balanced. These special feelings of LOVE and FEAR were used by the kind bacteria to keep them alive and to thrive and build in numbers as herds, flocks, pods and tribal families where they found safety in numbers in their harsh environment. They would fight to the death to protect each other.

The brilliant duo (kind bacteria and soft floppy cells) found unique ways to replicate what they had built by separating each species into two different body types, one male and one female; with specialist organs to produce half of the ingredients needed to grow an animal, bird, fish, reptile or amphibian. The growing stage could only start when the halves came together. It was so clever. Each offspring carried knowledge of survival stored in their DNA and each species found unique ways to incubate their offspring in a special bacteria free zone where even the kind bacteria weren't allowed. Birds, reptiles and amphibians laid eggs which were totally sealed from the outside world with the male sperm and female ova inside. The egg was placed outside of the body and the baby developed inside the egg. Animals carried their unborn in a special incubation place inside the female until it was ready to be born. The cleverly positioned birthing canal assisted the kind bacteria to take up residence inside and outside of the baby as soon as it was born to continue developing the child through its different stages. For example, developing the brain, nervous and immune systems, flora of the gut and protection for the skin.

The kind bacteria remained in charge of the symbiotic organism for hundreds of thousands more years using memories of emotions and feelings to control direction. At this stage of evolution there were two ways feelings and emotions could happen in the body. Either in response to life as it happened, for example, if a mammal roamed in the path of a predator FEAR would immediately happen as a response in the body to trigger fight or flight. Or feelings and emotions held in memory could be used to trigger a fight or flight response before the mammal

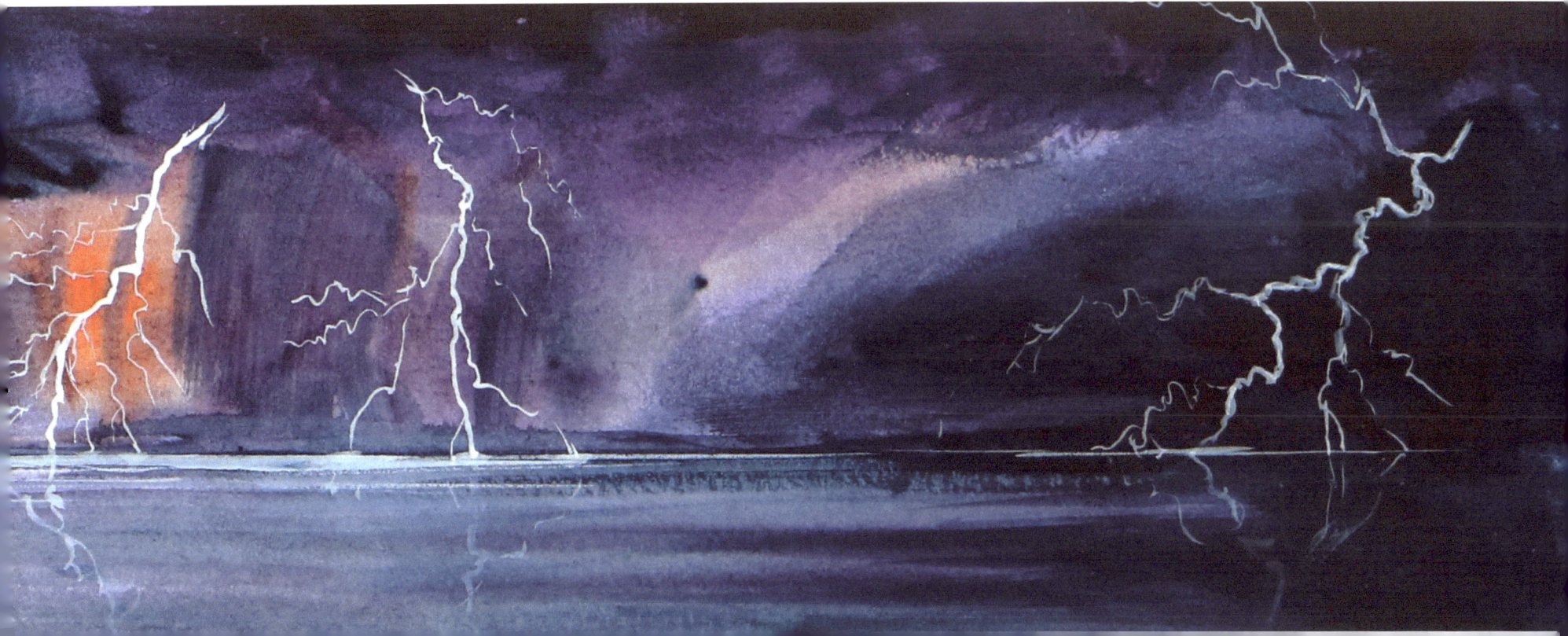

stepped into the path of the predator. Both used feelings and emotions to get the same result, however, one started in the body and one started in the brain. It was all made possible by the super information highways created by neural pathways situated throughout the body with links to the brain.

The soft floppy cells (now in the form of muscles and bones) had become jaded constantly living under the control of the kind bacteria. Whereas they fully appreciated the kind bacteria's constant vigilance to keep them safe, they always looked for ways to increase their share of control and waited patiently for an opportunity to branch out.

It all worked brilliantly well, harmoniously in balance with nature, until another species evolved – one that walked on its hind legs and had the power of thought which developed from language, constructed from words. This strange creature was the human being – our ancestor.

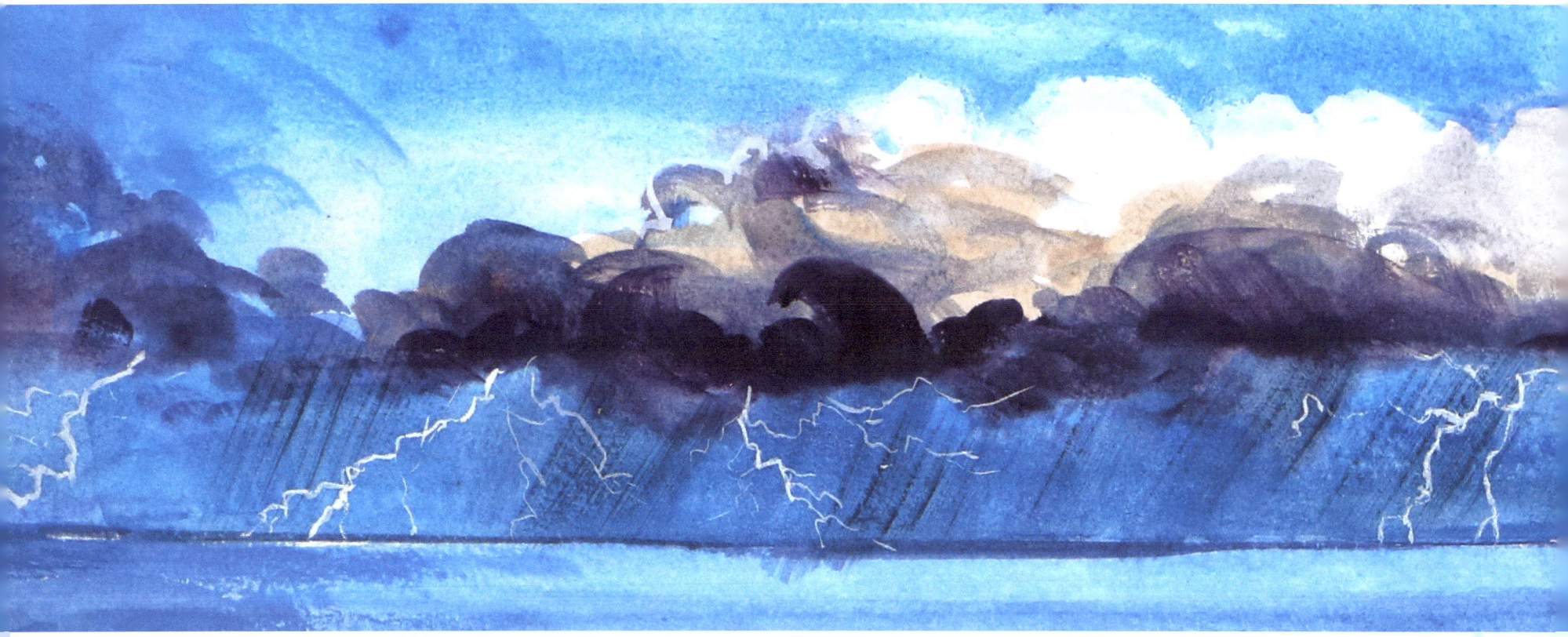

Scene Two – Language Opens New Frontiers

Balancing on two legs pushed brain development to its giddy heights, separating humans from other animals forever. The new upright position lined up the belly, diaphragm, lungs, throat and mouth forming the most perfect channel to the outside world. Wow, suddenly the body could use its vibrations to deliver all sorts of noises created from deep within. Noises that could be organised to communicate messages from one human to another. It was amazing! Exactly the opportunity the body cells had waited for.

Humans had survived for thousands of years without language communicating through a sophisticated system of sensory perception. A sort of KNOWING involving all the senses of smell, sound, sight, vibration, basic utterances and telepathic communication which could carry emotions and feelings from one person to the other. People were fully in tune with other group members without a word (other than grunts) being uttered; LOVE and FEAR radiated communication through their senses, delivered through vibrations and telepathically. These abilities are still with us today but not listened to in the way they once were. Language and sensory communication systems work simultaneously in the body and mind. However, the sensory system remains dominant because this is the system our two organisms have always relied on to keep us alive.

Language was built on words which extended the body's ability to send emotions and feelings to other people's body and brain. It was so efficient; the entire tribe could receive the one communication in the same moment. Even simple words like 'go there' and 'come here' worked wonderfully well to advance organisational skills. Words provided a new dimension of conscious thought inside of the person and this made the body cells very happy. Speech took off like a rocket – just like when we first discovered mobile phones! People became fascinated by their own voice which turned their body into a living musical instrument able to resonate a range of low, deep and high-pitched sounds. The round dome at the top of the skull amplified the vibration before it left the body through the mouth which put the final shaping into the words. The more people used speech the less they listened to sensory communication which weakened their connection

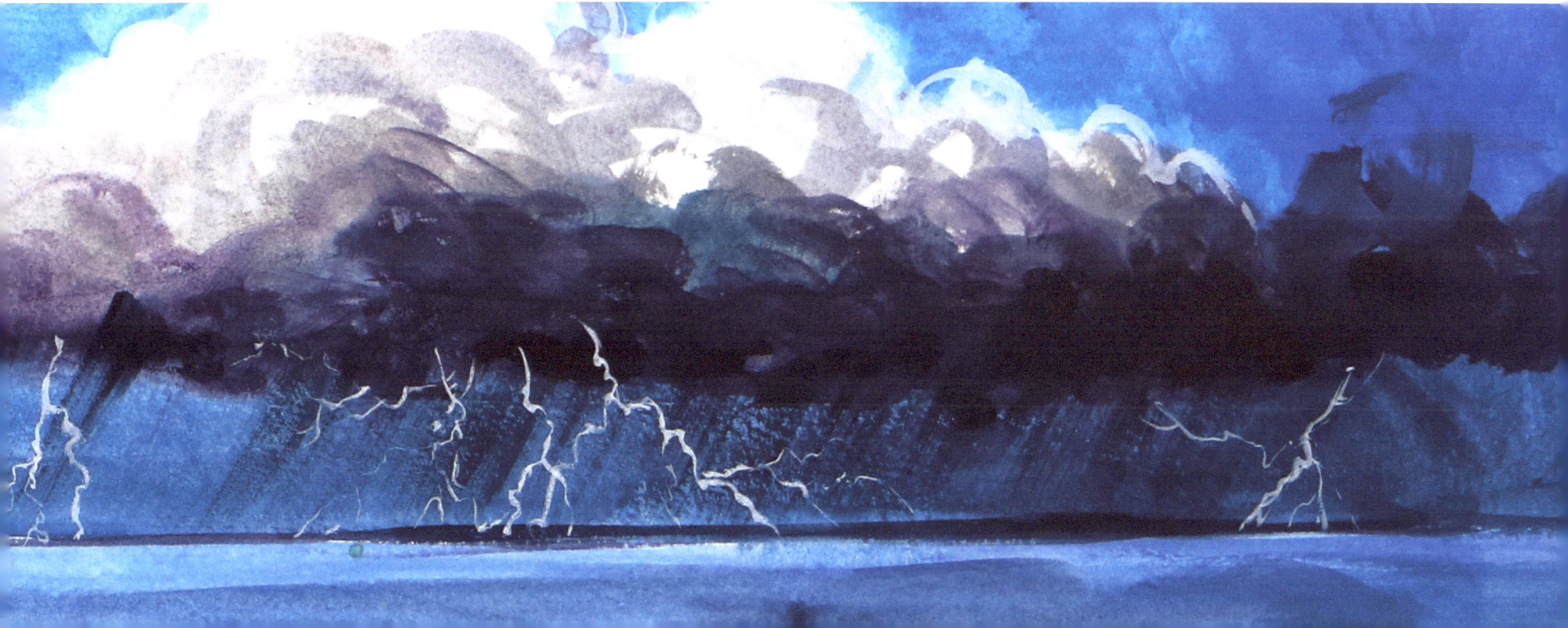

to it. They were too busy being fascinated by the sound of their new voice to NOTICE the subtle changes happening within.

More words using a wider range of feelings and emotions were developed by 'watering down' FEAR and LOVE. Those feelings and emotions that originated from FEAR triggered various levels of fight or flight while those originating from LOVE triggered various levels of relaxation. Or put another way, our feelings and emotions provide us with direction; we are either going towards fight and flight or relaxation. However, language slightly blurred clarity of meaning bringing a new complexity to communication. For example emotions can be used to change our tone, making it possible to use the same words to convey different meanings such as if I say 'I love you' with an authoritative tone it has an entirely different meaning to if I say 'I love you' with a soft and sultry tone and probably neither actually means 'I love you'. No one could predict the massive change language would bring to human behaviour. Before language developed people might fight for food or a mate but not over a simple misunderstanding. Sensory communication didn't require translation; it either conveyed messages of LOVE or FEAR but language using words carried a confusing mixture of LOVE and FEAR which had to be deciphered.

Quite a lot of unexpected problems arrived with language which evolved without a blueprint or a committee to scrutinise it. Hopefully this story makes us wiser to what is going on so that we can avoid unnecessary pain created by 'unforeseen design blips'. To keep clarity as we delve deeper into a complex subject let's introduce some characters to make it easier to SEE how our various parts interact and affect each other. The first batch belong to our bacterial side which has a massive variety of jobs to keep our bodily systems functioning. It's a bit like an ant colony where it's easier to identify the work and structure by job descriptions of Queen, workers, soldiers etc. As there are trillions of bacteria in our system we could easily create thousands of job titles, but our story only needs three at this stage and one other will be introduced later in our story. Those jobs are (1) fight and flight; (2) creating predictable behaviour patterns; and (3) the need to protect the organism from experiencing unnecessary pain. We'll call these three specialist areas Alerto (fight or flight), Habitu (habitual behaviours) and Oucho (protection from pain). Knowing about Alerto, Habitu and Oucho helps us to track the effect the newcomer (language) had on our symbiotic organism, which we call home.

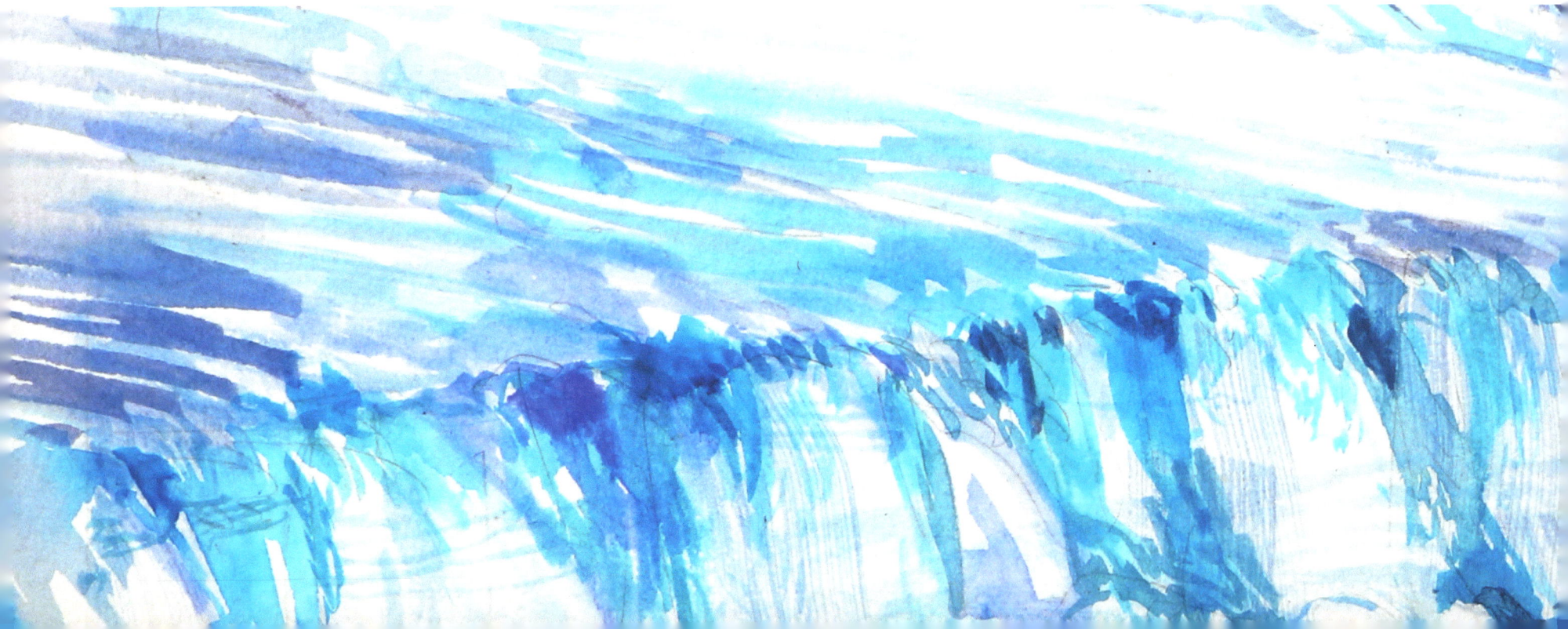

Problems created by language emerged soon after newly formed words carrying fearful responses were stored alongside 'FEAR filled memories' that Alerto used to trigger the fight or flight response. It's a storage thing isn't it? We usually do put 'alike things' together. Cans of beans go over there, and biscuits go over here! It would seem perfectly logical to put memories of emotions in the same place as words with emotions attached. However, storing words that contained emotions of FEAR near FEAR filled memories was a bit like storing the fireworks near the matches. Some things do need to be separated!

Suddenly feelings and emotions stored in words could accidentally trigger the fight or flight response. Unheard of before language arrived; the ramifications were ugly to say the least, opening a pathway to mental and physical health issues. It all started when our naive body cells first ventured into the memory to play with words. The moment they replayed a memory containing FEAR they accidentally triggered Alerto releasing a cocktail of chemicals into the body in preparation for fight or flight. Oops! The entire organism immediately felt the response, but the body cells had no idea they caused it. FEAR activated the mind which released a flood of horrible imaginings. Within a split second a full-blown panic attack was launched, without a shred of danger in sight. The

panicked mind set off on wild goose chases frantically searching the memory for answers but there were no answers to be found other than – Oops! I've accidentally set off a False Alarm – which no-one likes to admit!

Accidentally releasing fear overstimulated the mind;
which activated the imagination with wild thoughts;
releasing more FEAR into the system;
re-triggering the fight and flight response;
escalating the situation without a shred of real danger in sight.

The kind bacteria adored their body cells and could cope with occasional blunders but needed to protect specialist areas of the brain programmed to look after bodily functions such as running the heart and lungs; transportation of food and waste around the body; and keeping the body at the right temperature. The problem was resolved by creating a small sub-section in the brain where language could be developed safely in isolation; leaving the rest of the brain as it had been for millions of years – running on sensory communication. For clarity I call the isolated sub-section the 'Thinking Part' and the rest of the brain with its sensory connections in the body, the 'Knowing Part'. Data blockers were built into the

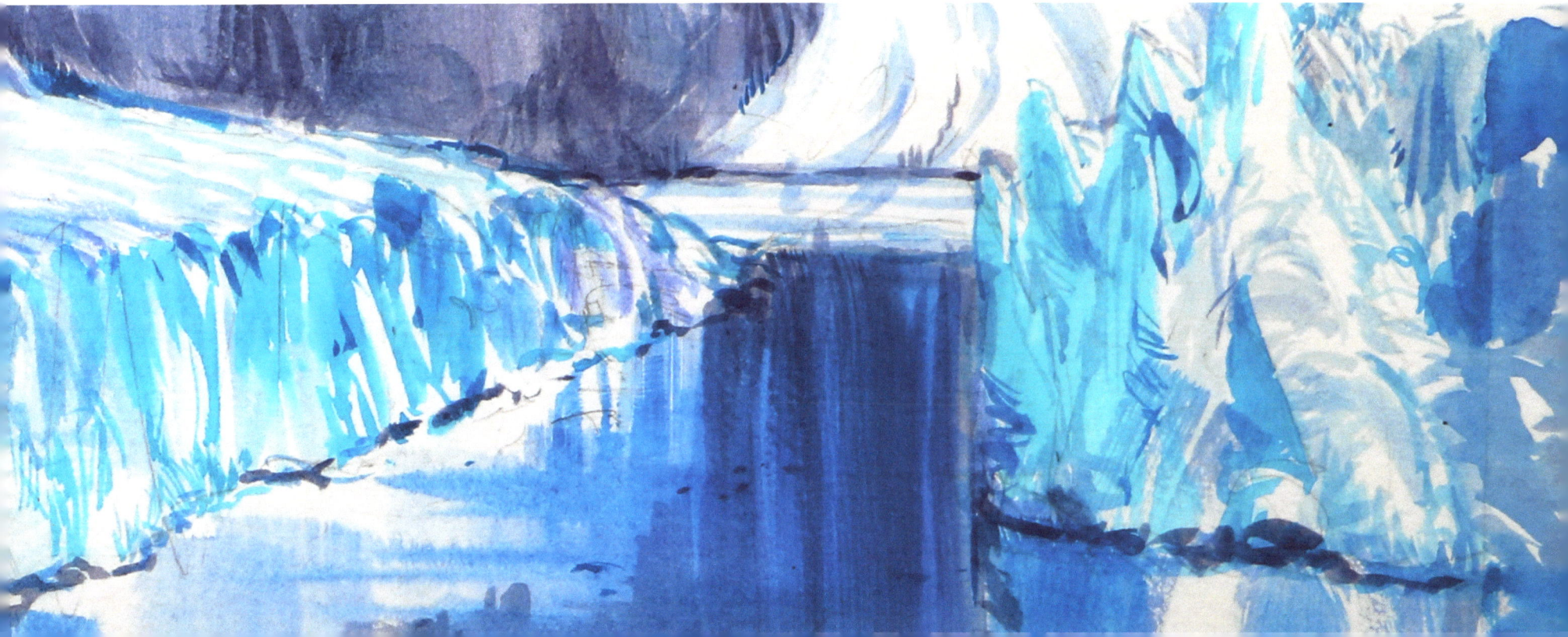

Thinking Part to prevent it being overloaded by unnecessary information such as billions of chemical computations necessary for daily bodily functions like breathing, digestion and body repairs. A massive amount of memory space was left, plus a few old memories as building blocks for new data.

The body cells were thrilled to have their own place in the brain (the Thinking Part) where they could mess around 24/7 learning to store and activate words, putting sentences together and gathering data without causing too much havoc to the rest of the brain. The kind bacteria (part of the Knowing Part) still had full access to everything and could get on with their daily work. It seemed like the perfect solution; besides that, what harm could the body cells do in a recording studio full of dusty old records? What harm indeed!

The Thinking and the Knowing Parts function differently and even feel different inside us. Basically, the Thinking Part thinks from within the head which is connected to the body; and the Knowing Part knows from within the body which is connected to the head. At first glance this could almost look the same, but it isn't at all the same. Two streams of information are being generated; one stream comes from 'known' information already stored in the memory and

the other is responding to 'unknown' information gathered fresh daily as life happens. Both utilise the head and the body differently but the point is they are both utilising the body and mind; this means at any one time we have two points of truth entering the mind and body. Truth of the moment and cleverly crafted truth designed by the brain to mirror the current event – which is not actually the truth but looks and feels very much like the truth. Both are recorded into memory as real events and both are important to our survival which sometimes might rely on our ability to run a pre-recorded escape plan rather than using up valuable time thinking things through.

The ability to re-run old memories was brilliant for multi-tasking, allowing us to do several different things at once, and for routine actions such as driving the car or doing the ironing which can be done automatically with very little thought. It's no different to millions of years back when the kind bacteria harvested feelings and emotions from the body and stored them in the memory to use later to activate the body before the danger arrived. Over time, this incredible ability became sophisticated, but still worked on the same principles. Once an action becomes known, Habitu kicks in and the action becomes an automatic response leaving our mind free to think of other things. Brilliant, but fragile

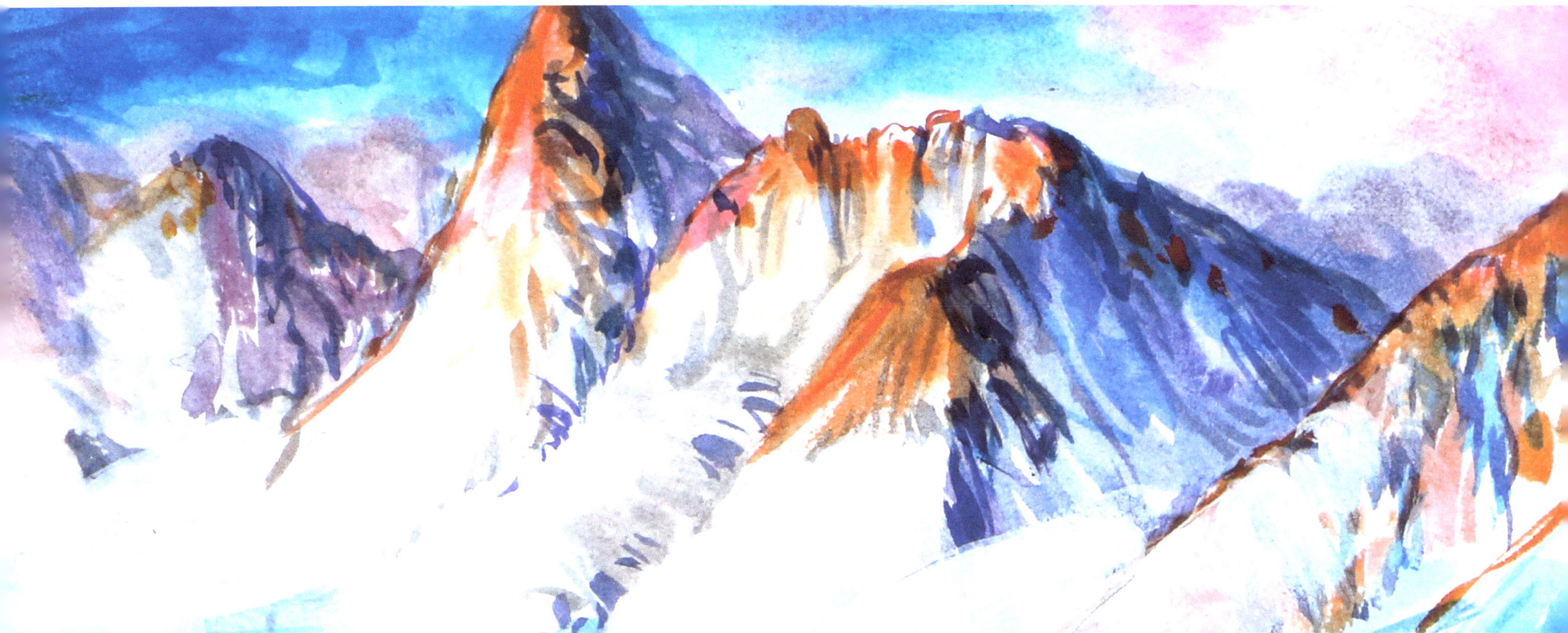

as it becomes extremely difficult for us to detect the difference between real incoming information and fabricated information manufactured in the head. We are left wide open to manipulation from our self and others. No wonder life and relationships can be difficult to manage.

Wait a minute! Does that mean we have more than one system of internal communication running through our body and mind at the same time without us being aware of it? Oh yes, it's like a radio with multiple channels to tune into. Our thinking mind only listens to one channel at a time because of the 'data blockers' but our brilliant Knowing Part receives the lot simultaneously because that amount of incoming data would 'blow our thinking mind' into oblivion. We need to remind our Thinking Part that it is only a tiny speck in a massive and brilliant system, but unfortunately because of its isolation our Thinking Part tends to believe that it is the central part of our system.

- The Knowing Part has been in place since the beginning of time; it's our information highway and central intelligence! It communicates with feelings, emotions, sensations, symbols, pictures, dreams and instinctive reactions. It's not affected by the data blockers, has immense capacity to manage

humungous amounts of information in lightning speed and knows everything about the entire organism. It can connect to pre-historic data recorded in the DNA of both the kind bacteria and body cells and knows everything that happens in and around the person's life second by second. It's telepathically connected to the outside world, knows every chemical computation happening within the body, knows how to heal the body if it gets wounded, replaces cells in the body, defends the body from internal and external attack and is directly connected to the gut – home to trillions of telepathic bacteria. The Knowing Part only runs on pure emotions of FEAR and LOVE, it always knows the truth of each moment and only ever communicates with clarity and precision. It is our most precious asset once we learn how to connect with its wisdom.

- The Thinking Part is home to all language-based information including speech, thought and self-talk. It's a relatively new development in the history of our organism and its knowledge can be crafted from a mixture of pure truth and fabricated truth which gives it the ability to fabricate information at a moment's notice. It does this to protect us, but sometimes this part gets out of control and starts fabricating truth to the point where it changes

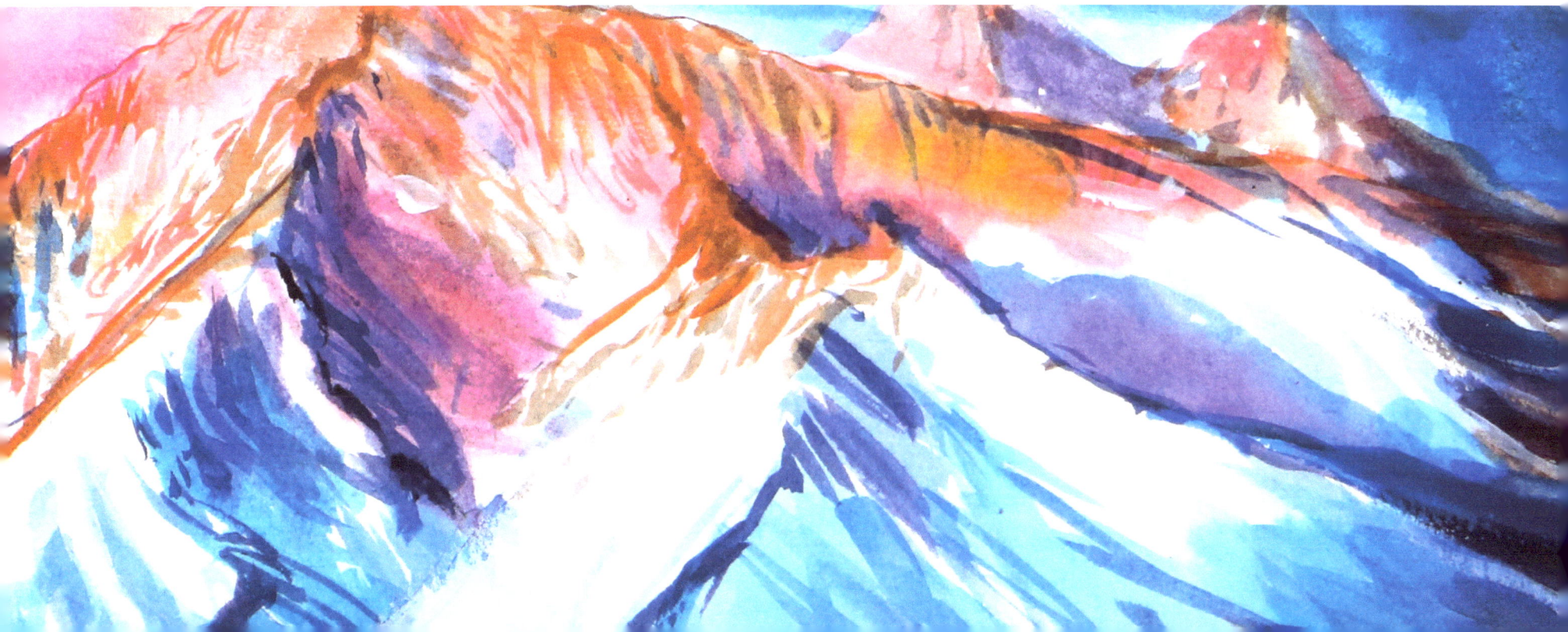

the person's ability to think logically. Language is much slower than sensory communication because everything needs to be taken out of memory and translated into words. The Thinking Part's main job is supposed to be asking questions of the Knowing Part and translating the answers which come without language through sensations, images, symbols, daydreams and night dreams, ideas and realisations. When the Thinking Part correctly fathoms the answer trillions of bacteria in the gut provide a gentle tummy rumble to let it know, 'Yes, you're ON TRACK'.

Wow! A system with checks and balances built in; access to ancient knowledge; fully in touch with the world inside and outside of the organism and fully in touch with LOVE in the body. The Thinking Part could even use the kind bacteria's telepathic system to send and receive messages with the world if it wanted to and attract things it wants. What a brilliant system. What could possibly go wrong? Yes indeed, what on earth could possibly mess up such a brilliant system?

Learning to think created a 'thinking voice' in the head which we call self-talk. Suddenly people could hear their own thoughts, which was weird at first, but

fascinating. People started spending more and more time listening intently to 'the voice within' paying less and less attention to their far superior sensory communication and gentle guiding rumble in the gut, always there in the background. Bit by bit, day by day the larger organism failed to NOTICE that the Thinking Part was forming a separate identity; its own persona. The persona (developing in isolation) had no way of telling it was just a tiny part of a gigantic organism. Two facets of the persona that developed are our next characters: one is our villain and the other our hero.

Our villain's character is irresponsible, arrogant and egotistical; doesn't manage feelings and emotions at all well and is either inappropriately 'up itself' or depressingly in a deep low mood. The more 'airspace' we give it the more arrogant and egotistical it becomes. Our hero is quite the opposite, very responsible, kind, sincere and considerate of others, knows how to access and wisely use all our feelings and emotions with great maturity. Please meet Arrogantio our villain and our hero Maturio; both belong to the Thinking Part of our brain and both are important to our survival.

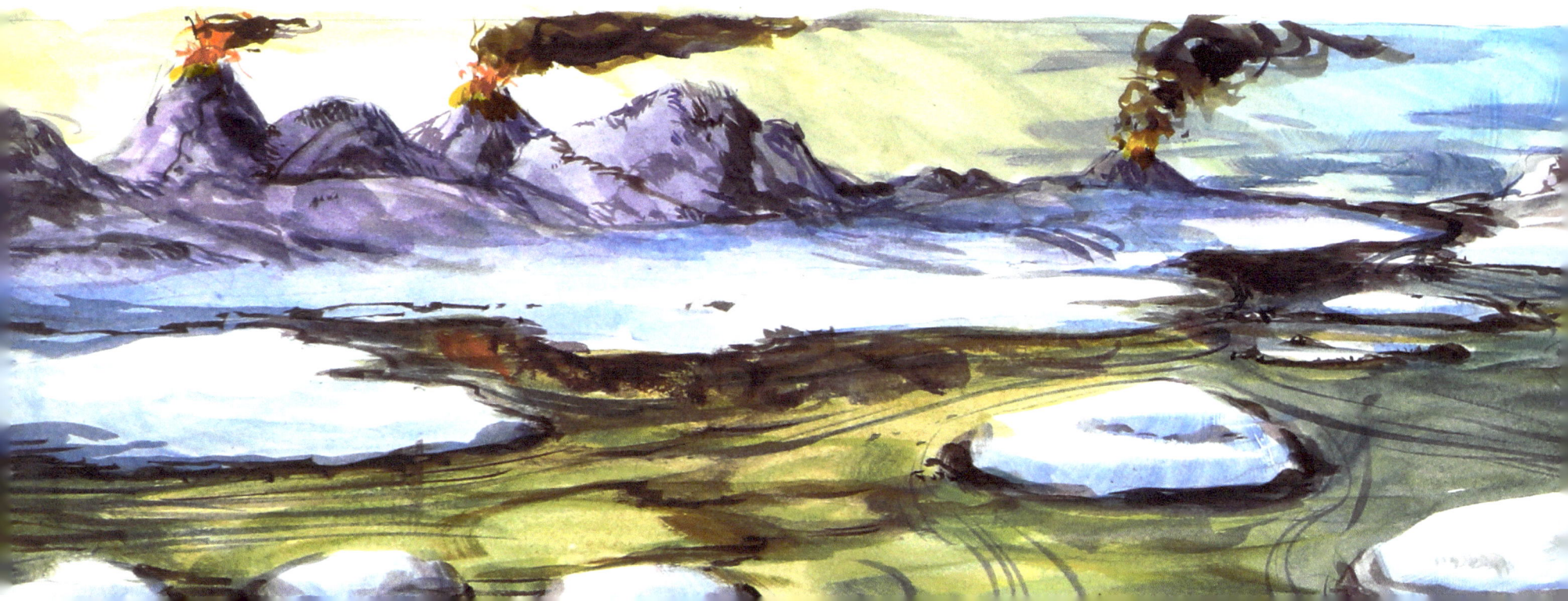

Arrogantio always tries to take over from Maturio, can be a pain in the neck, gets us into trouble and regularly wrecks our relationships because of its addiction to using FEAR based feelings and emotions to gain control. Arrogantio finds it extremely irritating and insulting to be told to listen to wisdom coming from the Knowing Part preferring to listen to its own fabricated wisdom. Let's face it, this does have advantages in that information can be shaped on the spot to fit any situation! Such amazing flexibility but Maturio prefers the truth and doesn't trust Arrogantio's tricky fabrications. It's a horrible struggle that has been built into every one of us. Arrogantio often becomes obsessed with its own importance and cannot resist challenging our kind bacteria who probably aren't even aware of its existence. Arrogantio brings a lot of strife into our life. Perhaps learning to manage Arrogantio is our next evolutionary stage.

It's quite normal for our thinking brain to fabricate information to fill information gaps because this ability is vital to our survival in emergency situations; exactly what it was designed for. However, not so good when Arrogantio uses it to fabricate information just to gain control. Fabrications are created from bits and pieces of memory randomly used to build a desired picture. A little bit of last Tuesday, some of last year and even a dash of make believe and tragically

we hardly notice and buy it as the truth, but our gut knows it's not the truth and does its best to warn us. If only we hadn't lost the art of understanding the special language of our gut! Fabricated information can be fun but not if we start using it to build bizarre belief systems that don't even make sense but impact our life. A simple example is people who believe it's dangerous to tread on the cracks in the pavement or something horrible will happen. There isn't any logic to it, yet it gets handed down through the generations. Everyone has a few bizarre beliefs, probably set in place in childhood. Our problem is Oucho (our protector from pain) blinds us to our dysfunctional beliefs and behaviour as SEEING will hurt our pride.

Arrogantio and Maturio lived in blissful ignorance within their isolated home. Too busy to NOTICE the effect of Alerto, Habitu and Oucho; more interested in developing language by shaping simple utterances into words with feelings and emotions attached. Grouping words into different 'word types' of nouns, verbs and adjectives which could be used to structure meaningful sentences. There was so much to do; developing language was exciting. The more fascinated people became listening to the head, the less they NOTICED knowledge coming from the body – our only source of truth. Eventually Habitu kicked

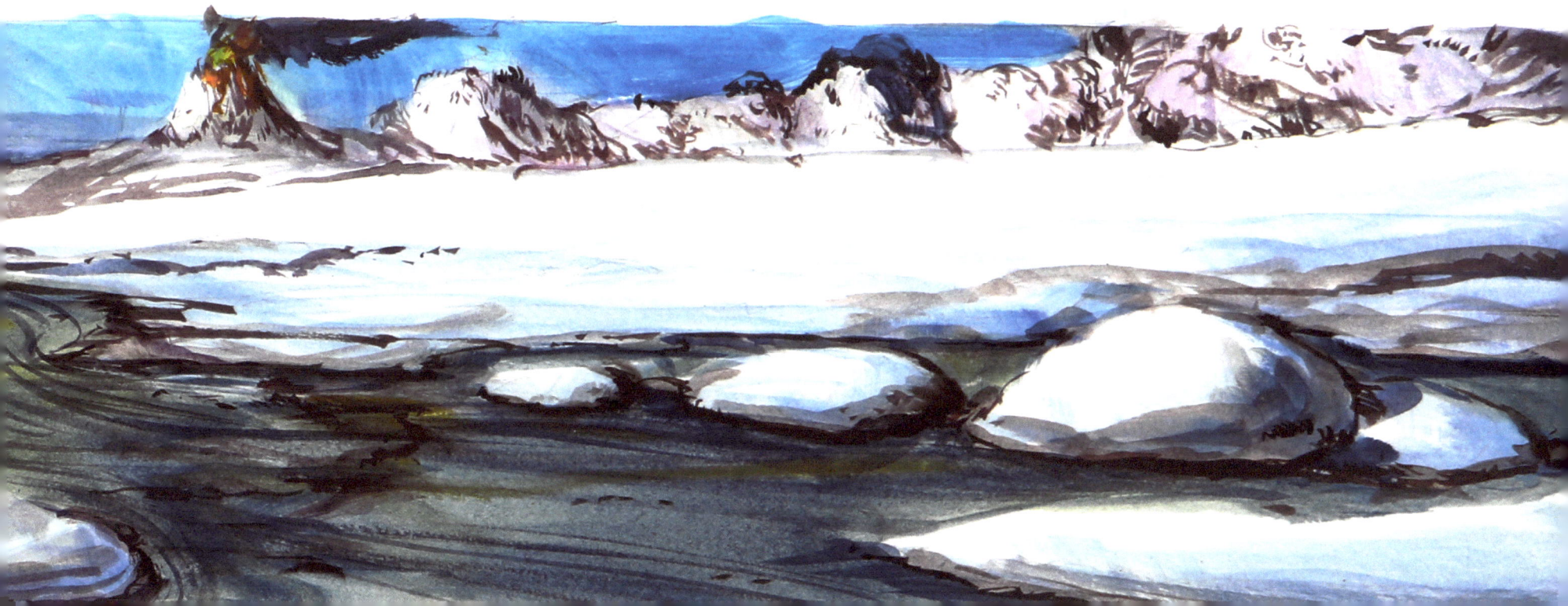

in to form a habit of trusting information from the head more than trusting information from the body. Many even forgot how to connect to LOVE within the body. It was always there but the connection had been eroded. Were people aware of this shift? Probably not but it was a significant shift.

Something new was happening. Our kind bacteria (Habitu in particular) had found ways to use language to hold us to predictable pathways. We didn't suddenly get an injection of language; it grew on top of our highly successful survival system, in times when our life greatly depended on Habitu's ability to build strong behavioural patterns, crucial to species survival. Language delivered much more power to Habitu's existing ability, expanding it to include habitual communication responses to control the direction of the organism. Just a few words uttered by one person and others could pre-empt the conversation and react without much thought. Fantastic thousands of years back but a frustrating habit today where so many people respond to each other without even listening. The response is trusted, therefore doesn't trigger any alarms, slipping neatly by, quite undetected by the gut and the persona. Our conversations go all over the place, we fail to NOTICE, then wonder what goes wrong with our relationships; quite unaware of so much of what we say to each other. Habitu also used pre-

set automatic responses to control the person, where certain words would trigger a predictable response – holding people in predictable conversations. It's a bit like family members who always say the same things to each other, year after year, with regular arguments that seem to have no end to them. We think we are in control of our thoughts however, so much about us has become a habitual automatic response.

The puzzling part is both Habitu and Arrogantio use language to maintain control and although the result might look the same it's actually very different because the 'intention' is different. Habitu is using language to protect the symbiotic organism and Arrogantio is using language purely to gain power and control over Maturio to feel big and strong. Our dilemma is we need to support Maturio by pulling Arrogantio into line, but we must NEVER step into Habitu's territory. How will we tell the difference?

Language also changed the way people lived in societies. Clever thinkers created rules to control the masses with disgusting consequences put in place for those who broke the rules. Our history books are littered with horrifying evidence of brutal punishments, prisons and grotesque public executions. How did that

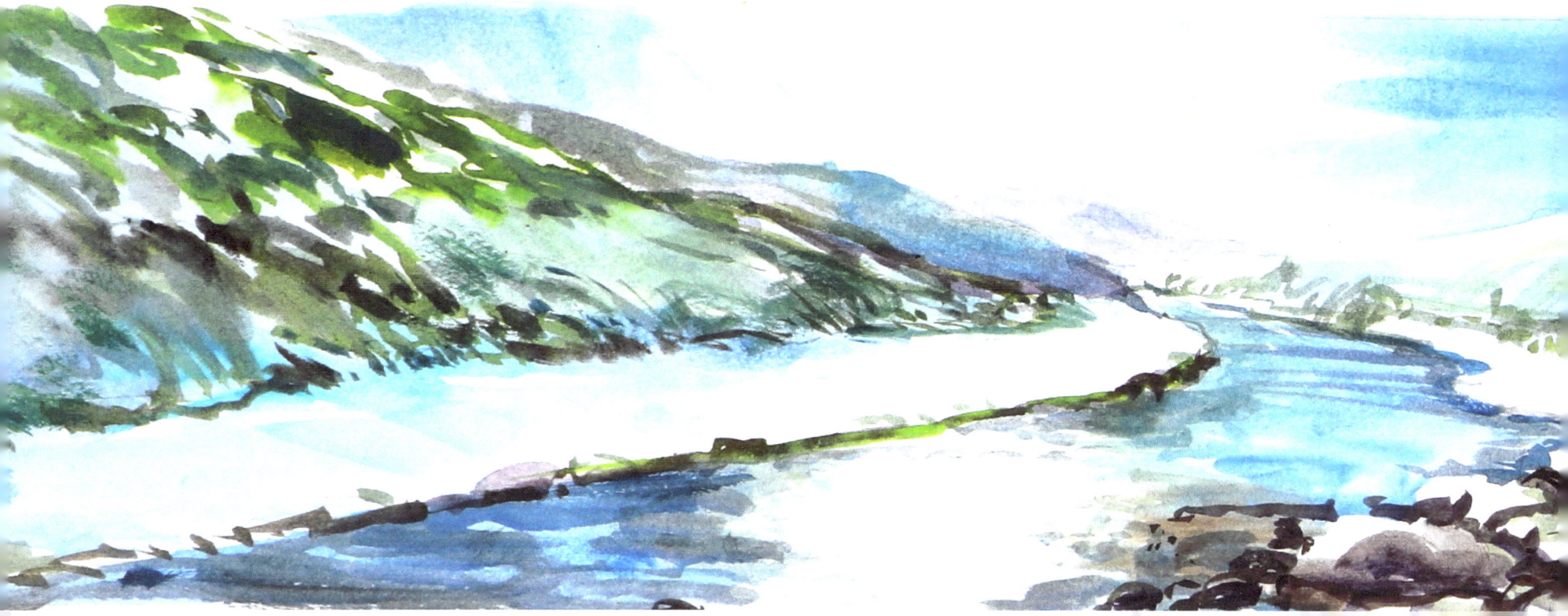

occur from a symbiotic organism built on LOVE? Obviously, something went wrong. On the upside humans managed to achieve the most remarkable things; building homes, creating food supplies and sewerage systems, information highways, electronic devices for every occasion, boats and trains and transport systems. The most amazing hospitals where people could almost be rebuilt. People even managed to physically leave the earth and send robots to explore the universe, but sadly only limited numbers knew how to live in health and harmony – experiencing the abundant supply of LOVE that is inside us all.

Can you see our characters at work in these people's lives?

Please meet Frank.

Frank was always nervous as a child and grew up worrying about everything. He lacked confidence and lived his life filled with self-doubt. When people tried to help Frank, he would become suspicious of the persons intentions. Frank's doctor has put him on anti-depressants and referred him to counselling – but it doesn't seem to be working very well for Frank.

Please meet Julia.

Julia was very bright at school; her marks topped the class. She worked so hard and rarely had time to play with other children. Julia didn't have any close friends to take home which was good as her mother was so clean and tidy that other children might have made a mess of her perfectly beautiful house. Her father was a workaholic and rarely around, in fact Julia didn't really know much about him. She thought he didn't love her. Maybe she was an embarrassment to him and she felt guilty about this. Julia grew up to be a top executive of a very large international firm, but she didn't really value her success. She had several short-term relationships but couldn't sustain closeness for too long. She worries about her inability to establish a long-term friendship. Julia uses alcohol to dull her pain, only the pain won't go away – so she keeps on drinking. Julia is clever enough to hide her problem from her employer.

Please meet Matthew.

Matthew is a happy go lucky sort of fellow. Everyone loved him at school. His mother made great lunches which he was always happy to share with others. His school work wasn't always the greatest, but he was a star on the sports field.

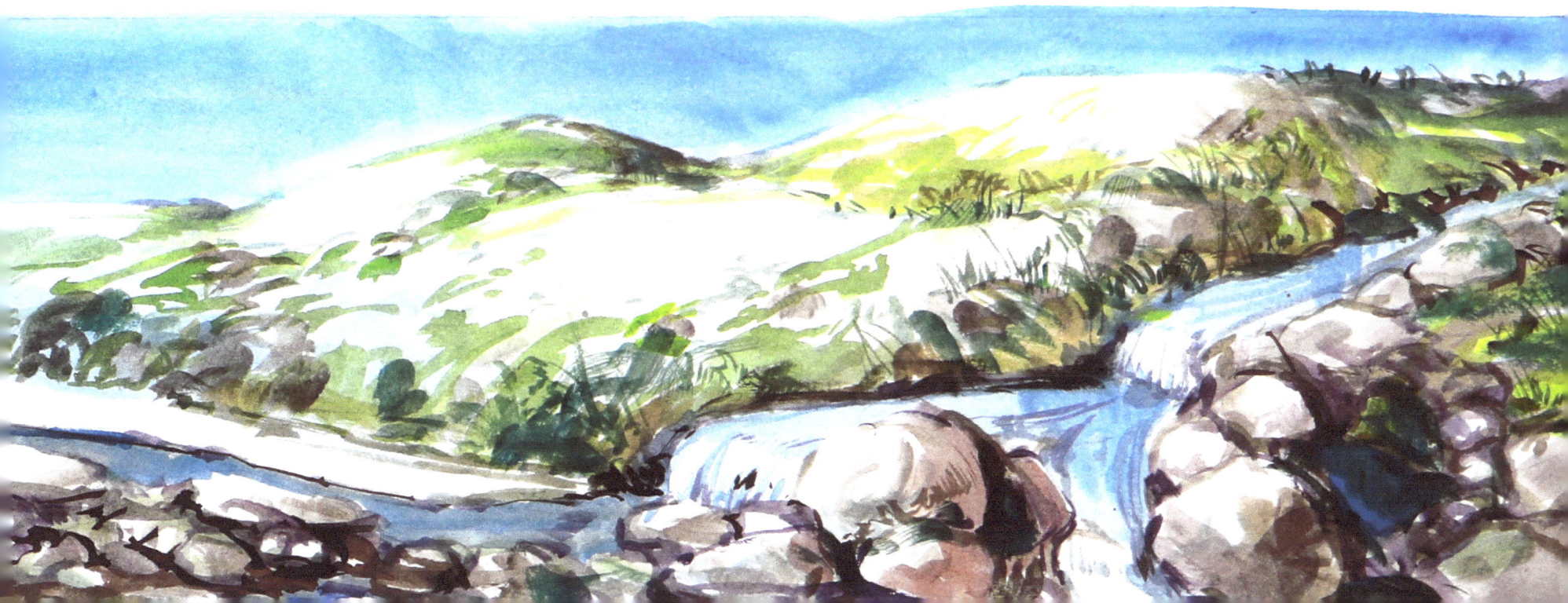

Matthew learned quite early in life that not all other kids were kind, sometimes he would go home in tears. Matthew's mother and father worked well as a team to give him great support. They taught him how to forgive and let go of the pain and get on with being happy. It was amazing how well he learned to manage other people and not be affected by their unhappiness and negativity. Matthew keeps up his fitness and is a loving and kind man to his wife and children.

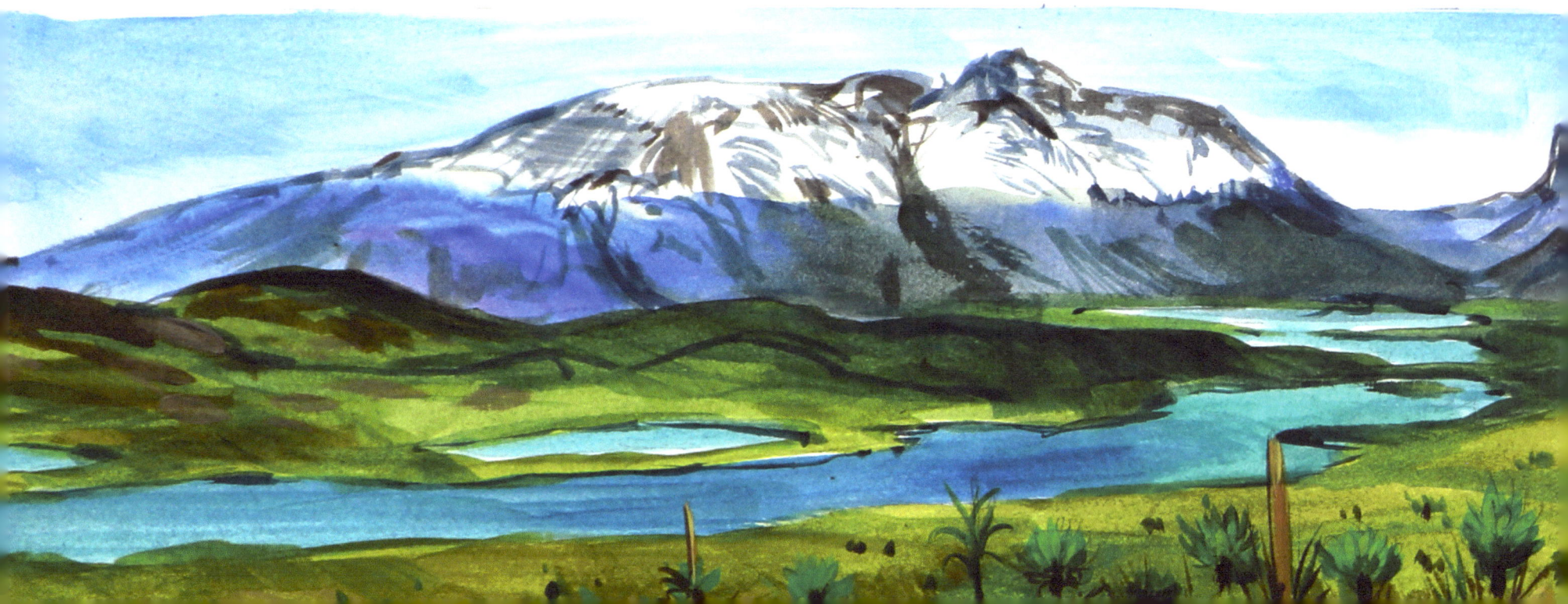

Scene Three – Our Dilemma and a Glimpse of the Solutions

From Arrogantio's view point (isolated within the Thinking Part) the memory was a wonderful playground full of words with recorded feelings and emotions with attachments to various parts of the body. The tiniest flick of FEAR got the most wonderful reactions; muscles moved, nerves twitched. It was thrilling to watch adrenalin pumping through the body causing the heart to race, lungs to heave, blood pumping wildly. How exciting; never mind about the poor person's Maturio being thrown into chaos and terror. Best of all, FEAR could immobilise and stop the person in their tracks or send them in different directions – like a kid playing with a remote-controlled car. Having control over Maturio felt powerful. It didn't take Arrogantio long to become highly skilled, applying FEAR in various doses from little trickles of fluttery fear to full blown terrifying volcanic eruption FEAR. Best of all FEAR kept that pesky gut so busy that Maturio could no longer hear the delicate tummy rumbles which appeared to challenge Arrogantio's 'superior' wisdom.

Unfortunately, Alerto, Habitu and Oucho did not evolve with the ability to detect false alarms as that wasn't needed before language arrived. Arrogantio had no idea Habitu existed and no idea that playing with FEAR for too long set a habit in place, creating a self-perpetuating cycle where FEAR triggered more FEAR. What started as good fun for Arrogantio ended as a horrible addiction to playing with FEAR. The results were horrific for humanity. Millions ended up with stress related diseases or mental health issues all because their bodies were responding to FEAR which had been triggered without a shred of danger in sight.

Arrogantio was left with an ever-growing sense of inadequacy and deep-seated terror but cleverly found ways to bluff a sense of safety to cover up the inner turmoil. Unfortunately, because the deception was based in FEAR it carried an underlying message of FEAR, blocking the release of LOVE and healing sexual energy. Sexual energy works like a tiny droplet of fine engine oil making sure everything in the body flows smoothly. It's very important to our overall health and wellbeing but has nothing to do with procreation and sexuality other than making our body fully alive and attractive to others.

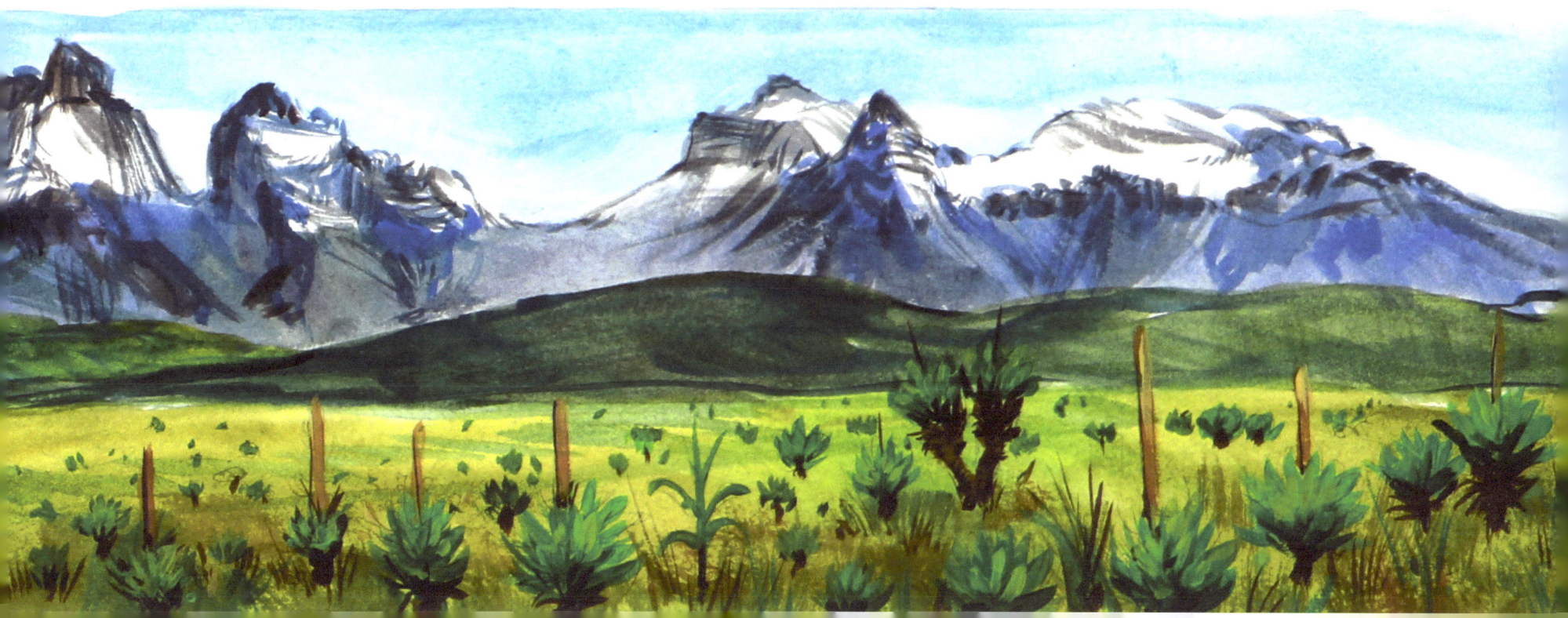

The more Arrogantio pretended to feel safe, the more FEAR entered the system creating an agonising cycle without an exit door! The less contact the person had with LOVE the more Habitu learned to distrust LOVE. Oh no! And when LOVE did manage to shine through with its familiar whoosh of wonderfully all-encompassing feelings, warm white light radiating healing vibrations throughout the entire body – Habitu fought against it. As senseless as this might seem if LOVE isn't experienced all the time, it will feel alien to Habitu. Is this a design fault? Who would know, but it can leave a person with a sense of emptiness – and even that can become a habit. Arrogantio counteracted by filling the person with memories of love, which worked in the short term but eventually left a deep sense of dissatisfaction and discontentment. Some people turned to bizarre behaviour looking for LOVE while others entered multiple relationships in quests to find love. Some invested energy into getting rich so they could buy love while others tried to steal love – but it wasn't anything like LOVE. People were left with horribly confusing emotional deficits; young children grew up regularly exposed to unbalanced emotions, which became the norm for millions of people. Quite often this led to acts of violence and sexual abuse within families, causing little children to suffer in their formative years. Robbing them of a sense of safety and setting patterns of abuse in place for the

next generation to cope with. Millions of people went on missions to 'find' their missing something, searching for answers in the strangest places.

People tried to make sense of the world from inside their head, and through libraries and heralded schools of thought. Life became filled with an abundance of 'not quite the truth' situations leading to disputes and unhappy relationships. People craved the truth. Justice systems rarely got to the truth; long periods of social injustice left thousands of families feeling despondent. Some lashed out, while others took their pain inwardly which wasn't the answer either. Some were filled with an unbearable sense of guilt until they found ways to 'block' feelings altogether, leaving them without remorse for wrong doings, which only made things worse. The whole sorry mess depleted people's self-esteem, eroded self-confidence and increased vulnerability to mental and physical ill health.

Lack of connection to the truth and too much fabrication is the perfect launch pad for all manner of mental health illnesses such as schizophrenia, bi-polar disorders and manic depression. Not to forget the creation of mind monsters appearing as full-blown hallucinations; nightmares, daymares with no way to tell the difference. Millions of people all over the world mindlessly agonise over past

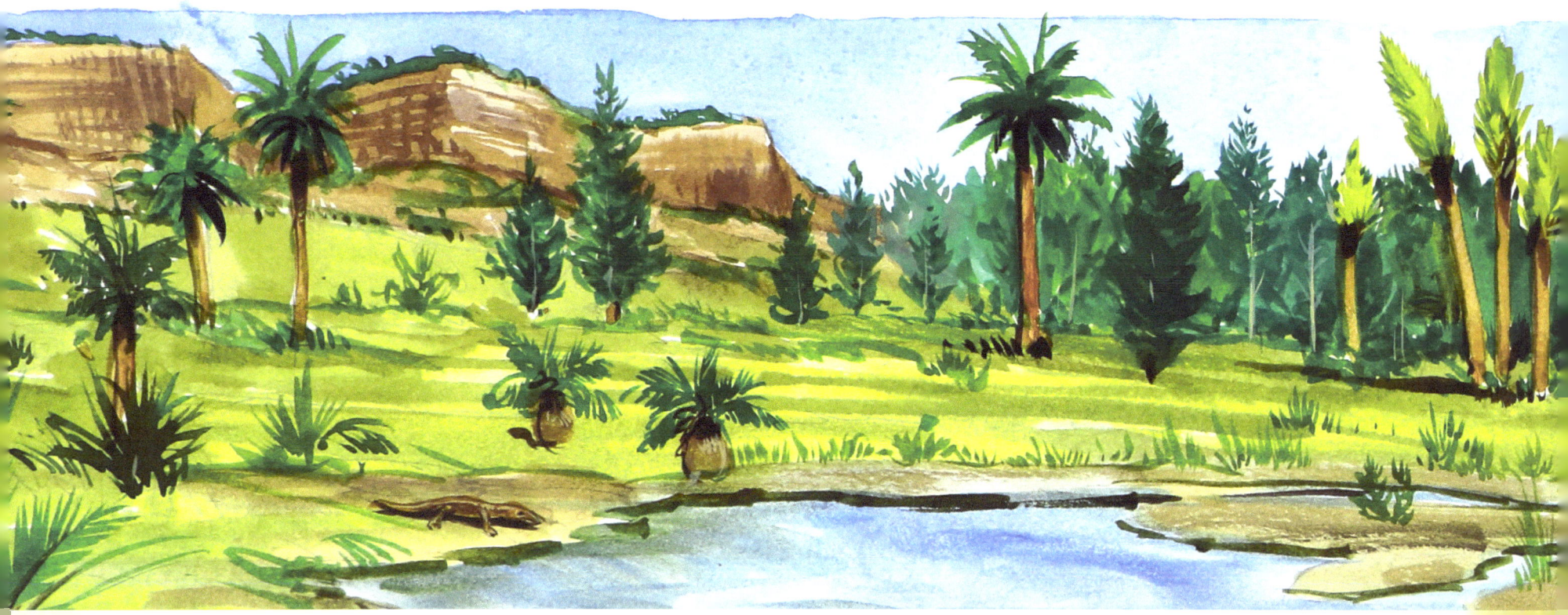

events, living in FEAR of 'what if' imagined events, fully addicted to filling every moment of the day with FEAR. There isn't a logical reason, other than an old memory containing FEAR is being refreshed; or used to build new FEAR filled stories. But why? Well, maybe Habitu has formed a habit of having 'horrible thoughts' and 'horrible thoughts' have become our new norm, locking us into tragic cycles of living in unhappiness – which we think is normal. No, no! It's just a habit which Oucho will not let us SEE to protect us from the painful truth. People rarely think to look inwardly to discover the origin of problems which keep re-occurring.

All sorts of professions developed around curing or healing people's ills; large corporations sprung up to create lotions, potions and pills to dull the pain; while others learned how to use fear mongering to promote, market and prosper financially from the sale of the pain reducing products and services. Advanced marketing techniques used emotive language and specific combinations of flashing coloured lights and beautiful body images to psychologically manipulate people to get the masses to 'buy'. Sometimes bordering on pornography just to raise sexual excitement; anything to make a sale without regard for how it affected people's health, children, or the society people lived in. The messier life

became the more governments and religions were inspired to put rules in place to control the masses. Even using social engineering through mass media to whittle away and reshape people's beliefs. None of it assisted people to manage their internal design 'blip' which continued to go unnoticed and unmanaged.

Habitu found so many ways to use language to hold people to known and predictable behaviours. Tone of voice is a favourite as it mostly slips by quite undetected. People spend hours pondering words, thinking back to what was said, yet fail to consider the tone used in the delivery. Vibrations in the tone give away the persons deepest truth. Arrogantio selects happy words to create the illusion of safety, but the truth slips out in the tone delivering an incongruent message. This is immediately NOTICED by our gut which sends an alert message – warning us of trickery and deceit. The gut is alive to the truth every second of the day. Its message comes with a sense of agitated nervousness which can easily trigger Alerto but that quickly calms down the moment Maturio gets the message. What a beautifully simple system. Unfortunately, when our life is out of balance Arrogantio overrides Maturio and works with Habitu to convincingly feed up memories of known events to provide a false sense of

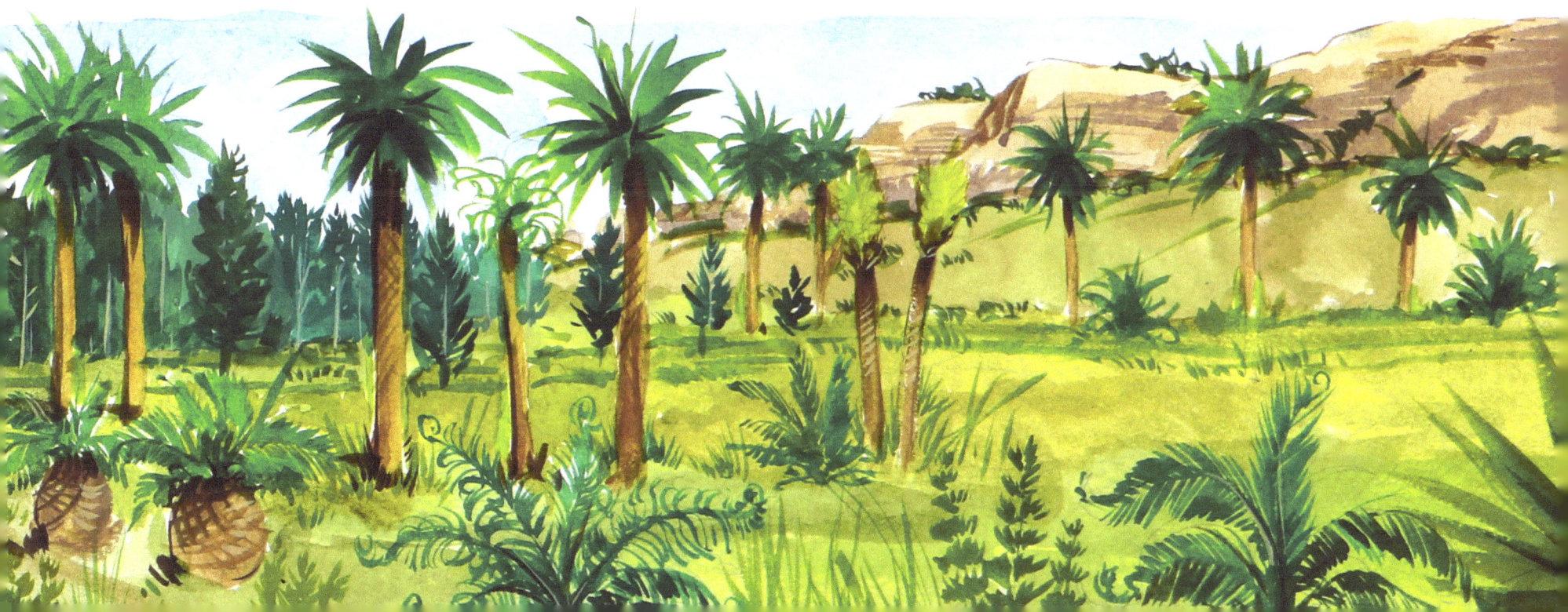

safety. We ignore the warning coming from our gut and we buy into pretend 'feel good' fabricated safety. Ooh! Not so good.

The underlying confusion sends our mind on relentless searches for answers when there are none to be found. Oucho kicks in to prevent us SEEING the painful consequences of ignoring our brilliant gut which is doing its best to warn us of deception. After a while Habitu kicks in to create a habit of 'searching for answers' leaving us on a merry-go-round. We have no idea of what is happening. Some of us become unstable. Surely this must be a glitch in our design! Either way, it's quite irrelevant as we cannot change how Habitu and Oucho function; they are part of our survival system and belong to our kind bacteria which has an entirely different agenda to our Thinking Part. The best that our Thinking Part can do is to learn to accept things as they are and find ways to work around Habitu and Oucho to bring our system into balance.

People who find balance usually glow with health because most of their life runs on truth allowing them to confidently relax allowing LOVE and sexual energy to flow freely. If some people can achieve this, then we all can. It all comes down to knowing what we can control and knowing what we cannot control, which

can be problematic if we start from a position of being totally out of control. Basically, we can take control of our Thinking Part – which is Maturio and Arrogantio, but must not mess with our Knowing Part – which includes Alerto, Habitu and Oucho.

Finding balance is the KEY to our success and there are a range of different things that we need to do to find balance. For a start we need to know the difference in feelings and emotions coming from our memory and those that come from our body in response to life as it happens. Once we can differentiate the two we can become selective of what we take notice of and what we discard.

'Memory' feelings and emotions are usually quite rigid, whereas fresh incoming feelings and emotions are fluid, moveable and flexible. Fresh incoming feelings and emotions leave us feeling slightly nervous of what may be coming next, which Habitu and Arrogantio don't like as they both want to feel safe and secure. Our gut (which is our greatest asset) relies on our ability to allow that slightly nervous feeling to remain because that slightly nervous feeling is our response to life as it unfolds. It's fresh and unknown. No-one can predict what is going to happen next because that is exactly how life is. When Habitu or Arrogantio

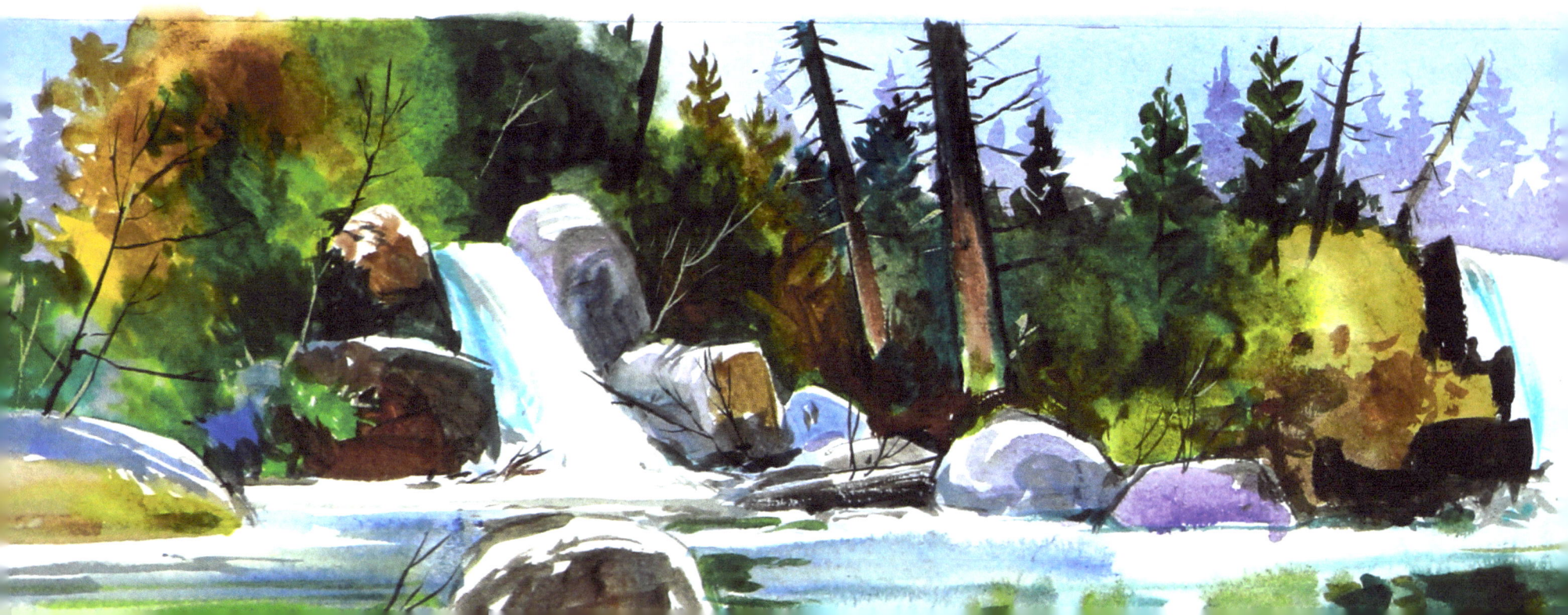

replace our 'slightly nervous' but truly alive feelings with 'safe' dead memory feelings and emotions, we end up living in a weird mind warp where old memories are revamped so often that we lose sight of reality. This definitely isn't safe but sadly it feels safe to Habitu and Arrogantio.

Ah ha moment! That's the crux of human problems; in our desperation to feel safe we destroy the very part of us that was designed to keep us safe. How tragic is that? No wonder Oucho works so hard to protect us from SEEING that ugly truth. 50% memory and 50% 'life as it happens' works well, but what if we're running on 90% memory and 10% 'life as it happens'? Pretty soon the blip in our make-up will encourage Habitu to only trust memory feelings and emotions, then we'll be in real trouble and the longer it goes on the weirder our life will become! Maintaining balance in everything that we do is of paramount importance.

A strategy to help us identify which feelings and emotions we are using would be to track our feelings and emotions along the balance scale. It can help us to SEE how often our life is being run on autopilot, using 'dead' emotions to respond to life. Even though looking might hurt our ego, SEEING releases us from self-

made traps. To use the scale, focus on any regular emotional response and ask: Does this response belong to the middle ground (balance), or the Submissive end, or the Aggressive end? Do not trust the first few answers as this might be Arrogantio's response and maybe we haven't learned how to tell the difference yet. Stay alert and learn.

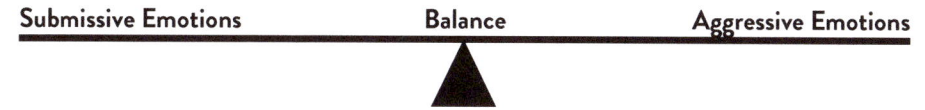

Submissive Emotions	Balance	Aggressive Emotions

▲

Ask: Am I in automatic response mode? Do I have the freedom to be flexible enough to move my feelings and emotions to any part of the scale? If we find we are unable to be flexible that is a sign that we are using memory emotions. They cannot flex as they don't belong to today. Trying to move them brings resistance from Habitu. Balanced feelings and emotions maintain a foot in both camps (Submissive and Aggressive) with the ability to flex in either direction to balance new situations as they come along. Living in the moment responding with fresh feelings and emotions which we use to keep our Thinking and Knowing Parts balanced. For example, if we meet a very aggressive person we can lean

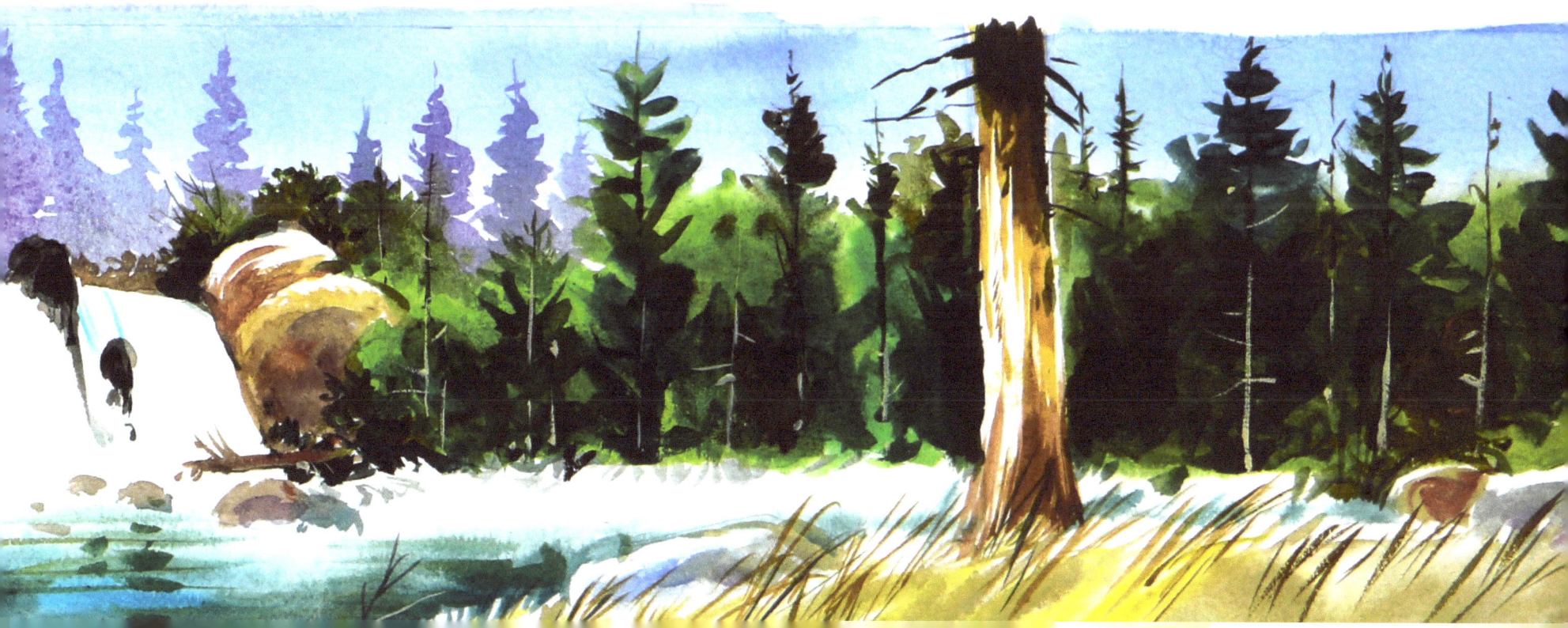

towards our submissive side – wanting to maintain balance by not adding fuel to the already ignited situation. Or, if we meet someone who is very submissive to maintain balance we might lean towards our aggressive side – not wanting to join in their despair. By 'staying in the moment' with that slight nervousness in our gut, we engage our ability to tap into our Knowing Part to sense what is happening, and our Thinking Part to choose our responses to divert attempts to control us. We remain balanced by actively experiencing the feelings and emotions that belong to 'our' moment while carefully tuning in to our gut for guidance. We use cleverly crafted memory feelings and emotions for our response. Our choice of memory feelings and emotions can be flexible, as can our timing, tone, volume; all of which affect our communication. These are the elements we need to experiment with when we want to bring change into our life.

Imagine if the other person is completely out of control, purely running on memory feelings and emotions, stuck in aggression or submission. We really do not want to join them in that space, yet they are actively inviting us in. We cannot control them; however, we can control our self by holding onto our space until they gain some control over their life. It's so easy for people to become 'sucked' into conversations where both end up responding in auto mode exchanging dead memory emotions. This isn't living, this is death without awareness. This is not communicating. This is thinking mind to thinking mind which fails to engage the whole person. However, if we deliver our response fully connected to that slightly nervous sensation of aliveness in our gut, we communicate from a position of being fully connected with all our parts. That's communicating!

If the other person is dead inside (cut off from the gut, living in cyclic patterns in their thinking mind) they may not be able to connect with us. They might reply with an incongruent response. It looks and sounds like they are communicating with us, but clearly connection is lacking. They are communicating with what they heard inside their head (cut off from their gut) and respond accordingly. That's the difference between communicating with the full self (head and body connected) and only communicating from the head (no gut connection). Our gut immediately alerts us to incongruence but only those who are fully alive will be able to hear it.

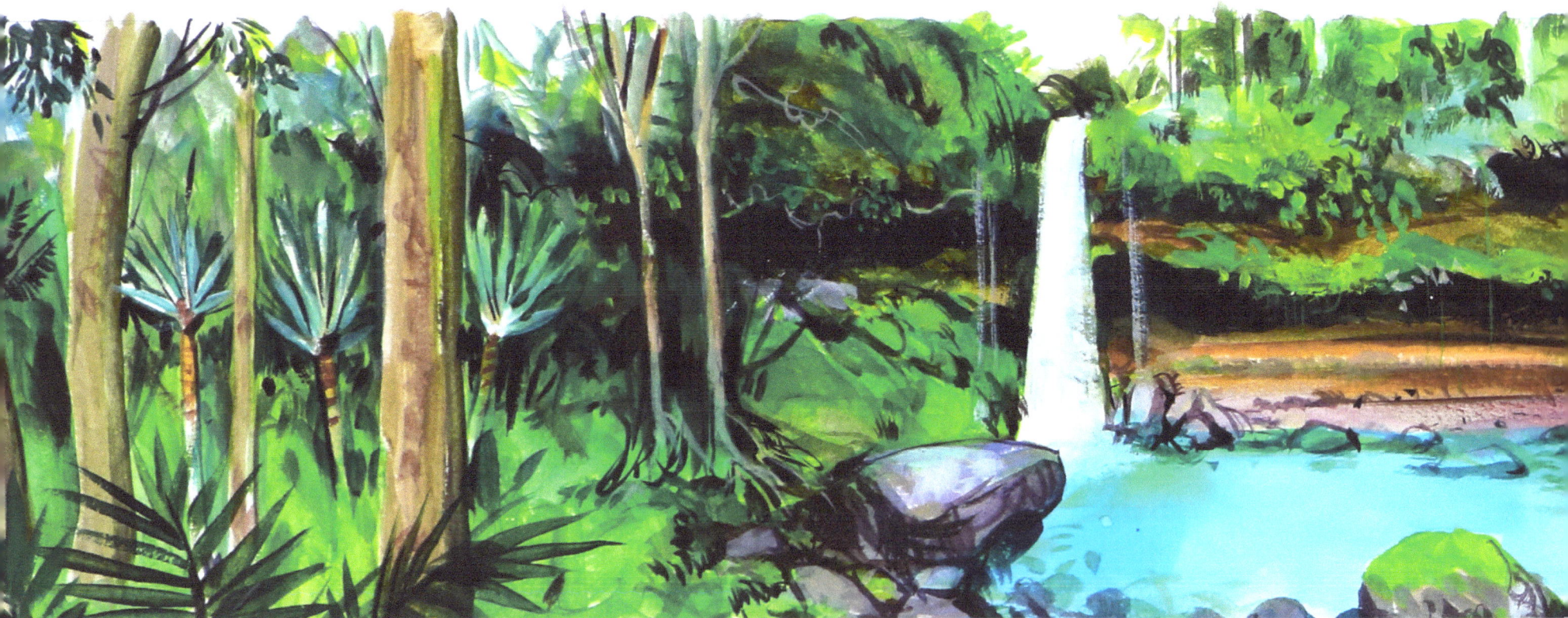

Balanced feelings and emotions usually lead to open and honest communication whereas unbalanced feelings and emotions tend to be used in attempts to manipulate and control other people. Being able to SEE what we are doing would be easier if we could look squarely at what Arrogantio gets away with; however, looking WILL hurt our pride. The pain of SEEING will trigger a reaction from Oucho, programmed over millions of years to steer our species away from pain. Functional before language arrived but in today's world leaves us totally blind to our own behaviour. Oopsie doopsie! No wonder life gets messy!

FEAR wasn't designed to hurt us even though it does feel horrible. But it can hurt us both physically and mentally if we get stuck in FEAR and fail to bounce back to LOVE once danger has passed. That's the big difference between humans and animals; animals do not hold on to spent emotional responses. The Gazelle gets chased by the Lion, escapes to safety and goes straight back to eating. The human would carry on about an event like that for years, hanging on to 'spent emotions', bringing them out of memory to refresh through the body, reliving the FEAR over and over again. But why, when the danger has long gone? What is the purpose? What if it doesn't have a purpose and is simply a

habit mindlessly held in place by Habitu because of a design fault (blip) in our nature? The fact is millions of people needlessly self-persecute for their faults instead of looking with kind eyes that understand much of human behaviour happens because of our 'blip'.

Habitu couldn't give a toss what thoughts, behaviours, tones or vibes their person becomes addicted to, as long as strong addictions are in place to maintain a sense of safety and predictability. Addictions hold us to predictable pathways and are necessary for our survival. Habitu is just as happy if we regularly exercise to keep it fit – or drink ourselves into oblivion – or keep thinking the same happy loving thought patterns over and over – or fill our world with defeatist negativity. Habitu simply holds the person to more of the same to form a predictable safe pathway so that our bacterial side can feel safe. Habitu doesn't choose the pathway, we chose the pathway and Habitu builds the routine. Predictable behaviour provides our kind bacteria with the best chance of keeping their home safe. They have no other interest in us, which means we are free to choose our habits. We just need to replace old habits carefully by slowly building new ones alongside them to avoid upsetting Habitu and triggering Alerto.

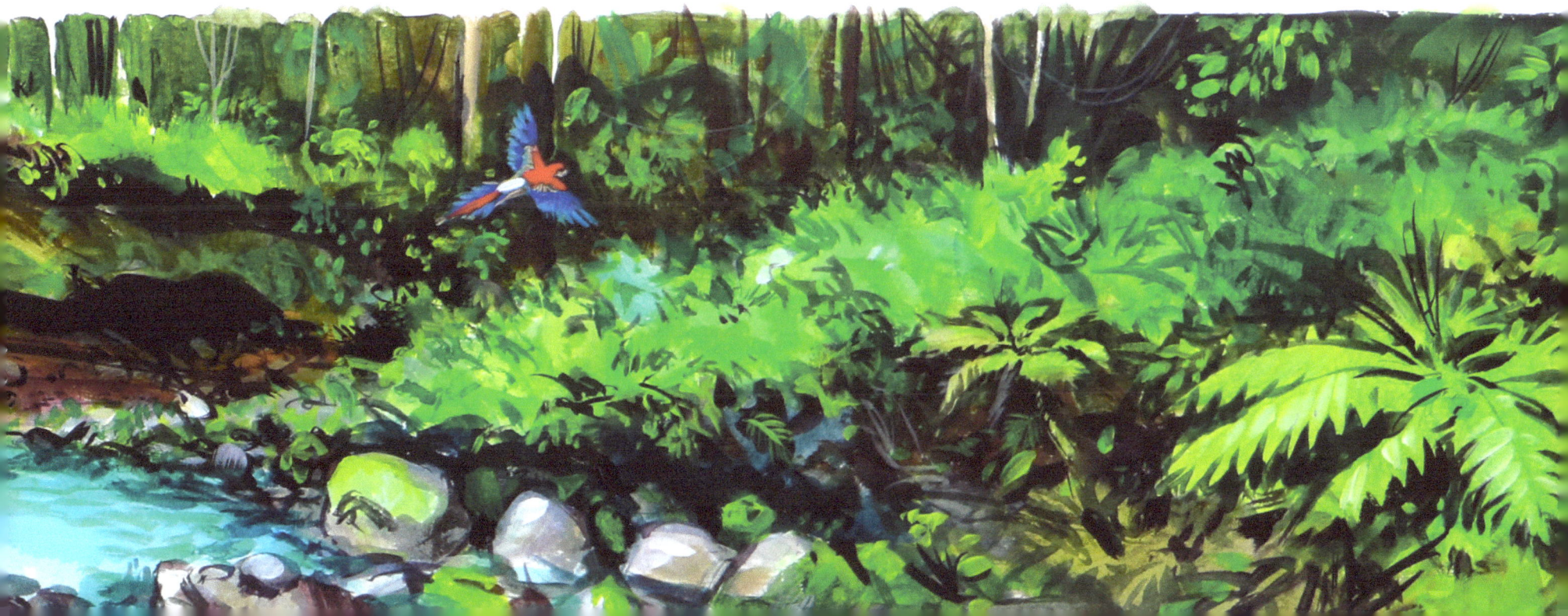

Our bacterial side does not have a master plan other than protecting their home. They are not one bit interested in our happiness or our quality of life. Better for us to come to terms with that fact as quickly as we can. Stop wasting precious time trying to change the unchangeable; move on to managing the manageable. Our life changes dramatically the moment we make a deep cellular decision (made within the cells of our body and not within the mind) to encourage Maturio to come forward. Part of what we need to do is severely reduce Arrogantio's air space and that is something Maturio needs to master. Yes, but even that requires us to be balanced and to have the ability to be assertive without landing back into aggressive or submissive thinking. It can be tricky, especially if we carry some life damage, which most of us do!

Okay, we begin to SEE how complicated human life can be:

- Alerto kicks in with fight or flight if it senses any sort of danger;
- Habitu creates addictions that have predictable outcomes just to feel safe;
- Oucho guides us away from pain to keep us safe – but leaves us blind to the truth;

- Arrogantio plays tricks, fabricates information, triggers false alarms and hides its cowardice by feeding us information that is not the truth, and gains power from keeping our system out of balance.
- Maturio needs our support to regain territory from Arrogantio so that our system can regain balance.

Well that is amazing. At least we can now SEE what we are dealing with. Here's another opportunity to see our characters at work.

Please meet Zanna

Zanna is a complex person who suffers from mood swings. It's hard to know where she is coming from and sometimes conversations quickly become complex and I'm left wondering what I have done to cause the change in her. I love her to bits but being her friend is really hard work. It's as though I trigger her black moods in the middle of my conversations and this makes me trouble over what I might have said. It doesn't matter how careful I am, I just end up walking on eggshells around her so as not to set her off into unhappiness. She scares me when she goes into her low moods because she appears to go into a very dark place and I don't feel I can reach her. I am so afraid for her and sometimes

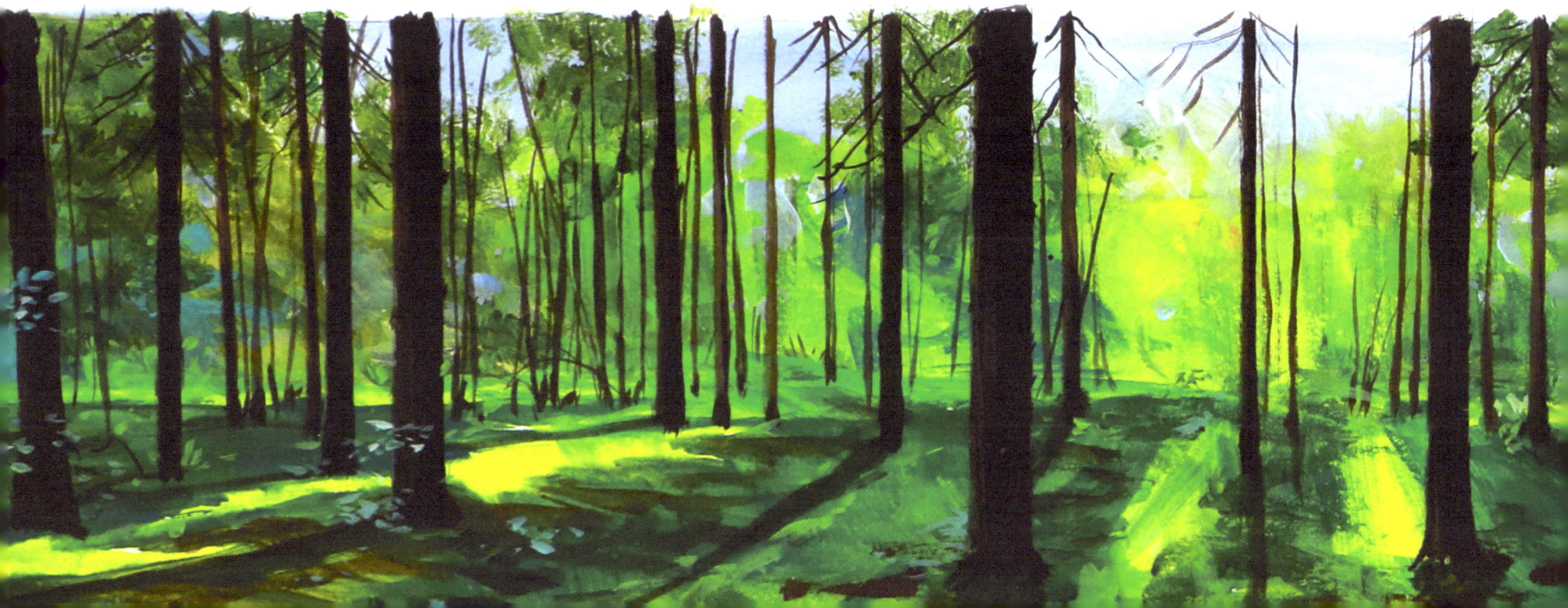

I'm afraid of her. She refuses to get help and says she doesn't have a problem because it's the people around her that have problems. I have no idea how to help and don't like to let her go as my friend. In fact, I feel a bit responsible to look after her.

Please meet James

James has two names, one is his Australian name and one is his traditional tribal name – but I only know him as James. He is such a lovely person, but he carries the weight of his lost nation on his shoulders. Sometimes he is consumed with rage and drinks too much alcohol. I stay well away when he is like that; he goes into such a dark place and doesn't want to know me. Then he pops back into my life as a happy person again, but his mood swings are not like Zanna's mood swings. His are way deeper – like a deep mourning within, a loss that cannot be replaced. Poor James has developed diabetes and heart problems and I'm very worried about his future.

Please meet Isabella

Isabella's family migrated to Australia years ago from Lebanon – I think they fled from war and arrived with nothing – only the clothes on their back. Life was very hard at first. Isabella's family had to put up with nasty racist jokes – but they found a way to ignore them and get on with their new opportunity in a land where they were safe from physical harm. Her family held at its heart the value of fairness which helped them to rise above all the ugly comments. Slowly the family became accepted in the community – her father got a really good job and earned enough money to buy a good home. All the children did well at school encouraged by their mother to rise above the daily taunts. The family keep their focus on the important parts of life and ignore the rest.

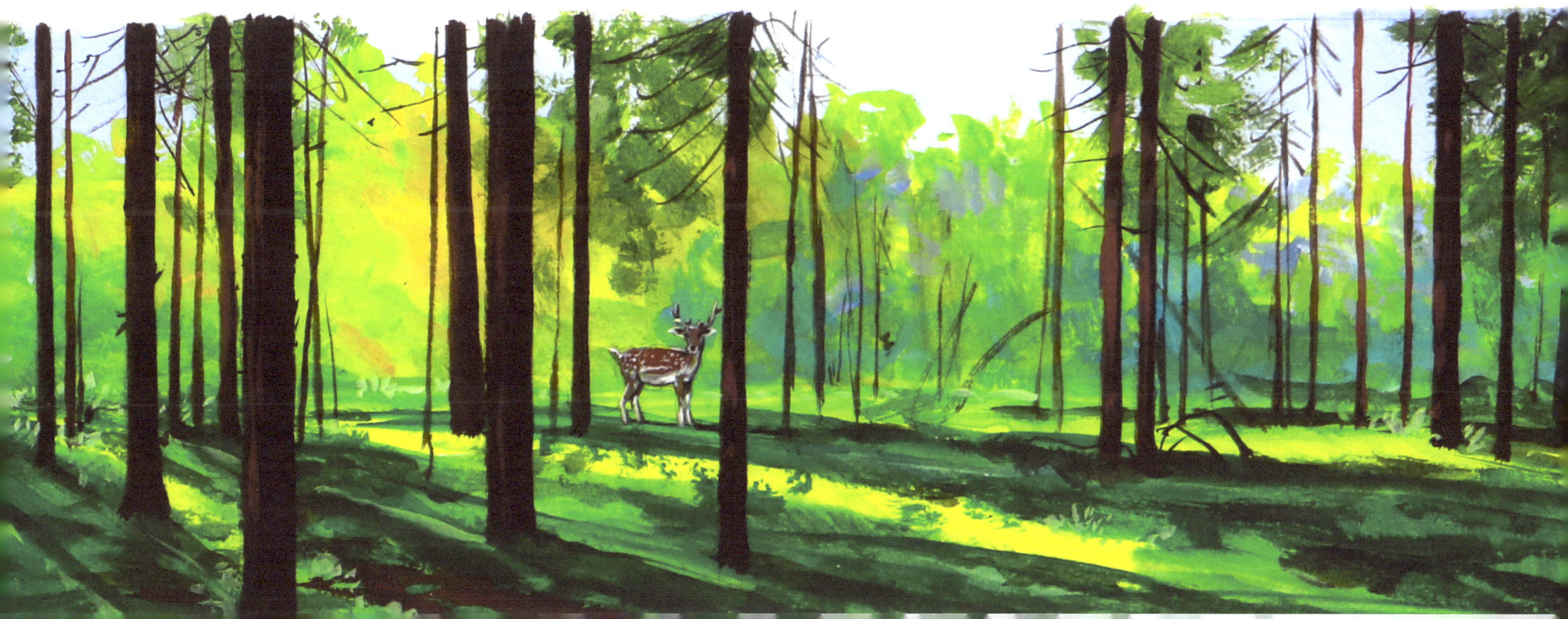

Scene Four – Removing Blockages To Brilliance

Balance brings our body into rhythm with life so that we function at our very best. For example, when balance restores between LOVE and FEAR a relieved vibration ripples throughout our organism as our bacteria sigh in relief now that our Thinking Part has stopped setting off false alarms. Our gut was desperately trying to signal us, but we were deaf and failed to NOTICE a massive part of our system labouring under needless pressure. Now our body can fully relax and reconnect to the natural flow of LOVE inside, releasing sexual energy to flow through our body, keeping everything working 'just right'.

Fantastic, but how do we get there? Yes well, there are many steps that need to happen. Most importantly Maturio needs to discover what the Thinking Part unwittingly does to upset the Knowing Part; accidentally setting up dysfunctional habits, which Habitu holds in place. These dysfunctional cycles, made possible by language, bounce endlessly between our parts and sit at the base of all human problems. For the Knowing Part dysfunctional behavioural patterns are something of an annoying buzzy fly, but for the Thinking Part this

can be the difference between a life of mental torture and a life of peace and tranquility.

Our Thinking Part needs to do whatever it takes to find balance because our symbiotic organism doesn't care as it copes well whether we are mentally deranged or stable. Maturio has some hidden talents to reduce dysfunctional behaviours. However, before Maturio can work magic it has to know where its boundaries are; know what it can and cannot achieve; know how to respectfully communicate with the Knowing Part; and know when not to interfere. Our greatest challenge is that Maturio and Arrogantio are two sides of the one entity within us, which means either Maturio is at the fore or Arrogantio is at the fore. We cannot achieve balance while Arrogantio is to the fore as Arrogantio's character closes communication with our Knowing Part. Keeping Maturio forward is a tough job until we change some of our addictions.

Dysfunctional behaviour cycles raise a small amount of FEAR in the gut, just enough to automatically over-ride LOVE in readiness to launch fight or flight.

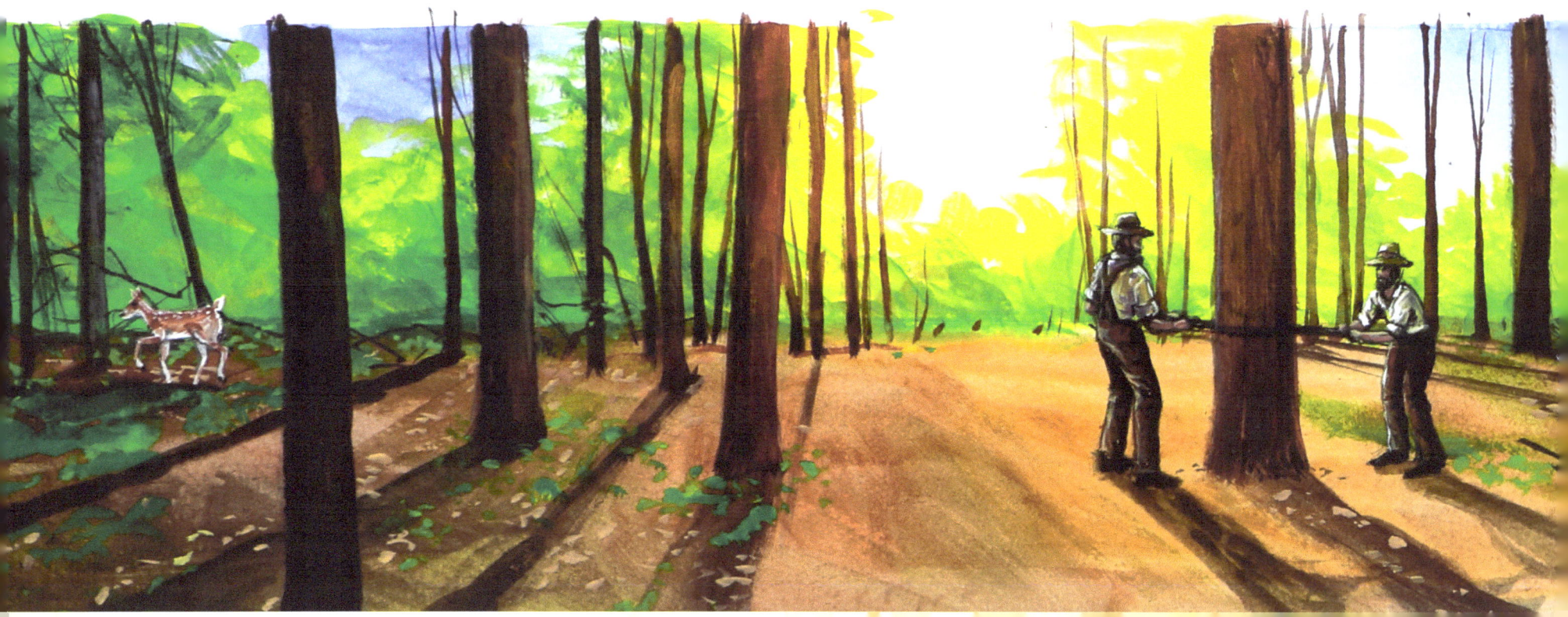

The small amount of FEAR isn't enough to raise our concern and slips by quite undetected, leaving millions unaware of the loss of connection to LOVE. The slow seeping loss left us unaware that the situation needed correction. Millions of people were left carrying an undetected backlog of old resentments and negative emotions, which wasn't part of our original design. We were designed to bounce from FEAR back to LOVE which floods our system with truth and autocorrects our daily errors, clearing unfinished business.

That's a lot to put right. Thankfully this task is within our capacity as our system is fully equipped with everything we need, once Maturio learns how to turn it all around by dissolving our blockage to brilliance. Our gut is our built in early warning detector. A radar to incoming danger which can pick up the tiniest deception in a flash. It's our fail safe and even warns us when Habitu is running on false information causing unnecessary FEAR in our system. How come we lost the art of listening to our body when it always knows the truth? Our gut wants us to get back to experiencing LOVE so that it can live in a relaxed and peace filled state. By learning to trust it and listen to its advice, Maturio will be led in the right direction to find balance.

When our Thinking and Knowing Parts are balanced truth floods in and amazing things happen. Our mind creates new neural pathways connecting pockets of knowledge stored haphazardly, connecting information and clearing muddled thinking. Light bulbs flash in realisation as old information is refreshed and revitalised. For a little while the brain aches from excessive activity as it restores and tidies our internal filing system. The dust and gloom are lifted from our mind and our thought processes are left clean, clear and uncluttered. We think differently, Maturio is less likely to become trapped by Arrogantio's tricks, making it safe to use our special abilities more productively. We are free to use our special ability to run movies in our head to practice different situations that we might find our self in and test different emotional responses in the safety of our 'play area' to see if it works without upsetting our bacterial side. We can practice 'back off' strategies and stockpile prepared responses in our imagination waiting for the right opportunity to deploy them. What a brilliant system! None of it would be possible without our ability to use memory feelings and emotions. Our system is so amazing once we get it working for us and not against us. We can use our imagination to change ugly memories and defuse old emotional pain. Who would want to be without such a fabulous gift; we can even 'act out' missing parts of our life to fill gaps in our experience if we want to.

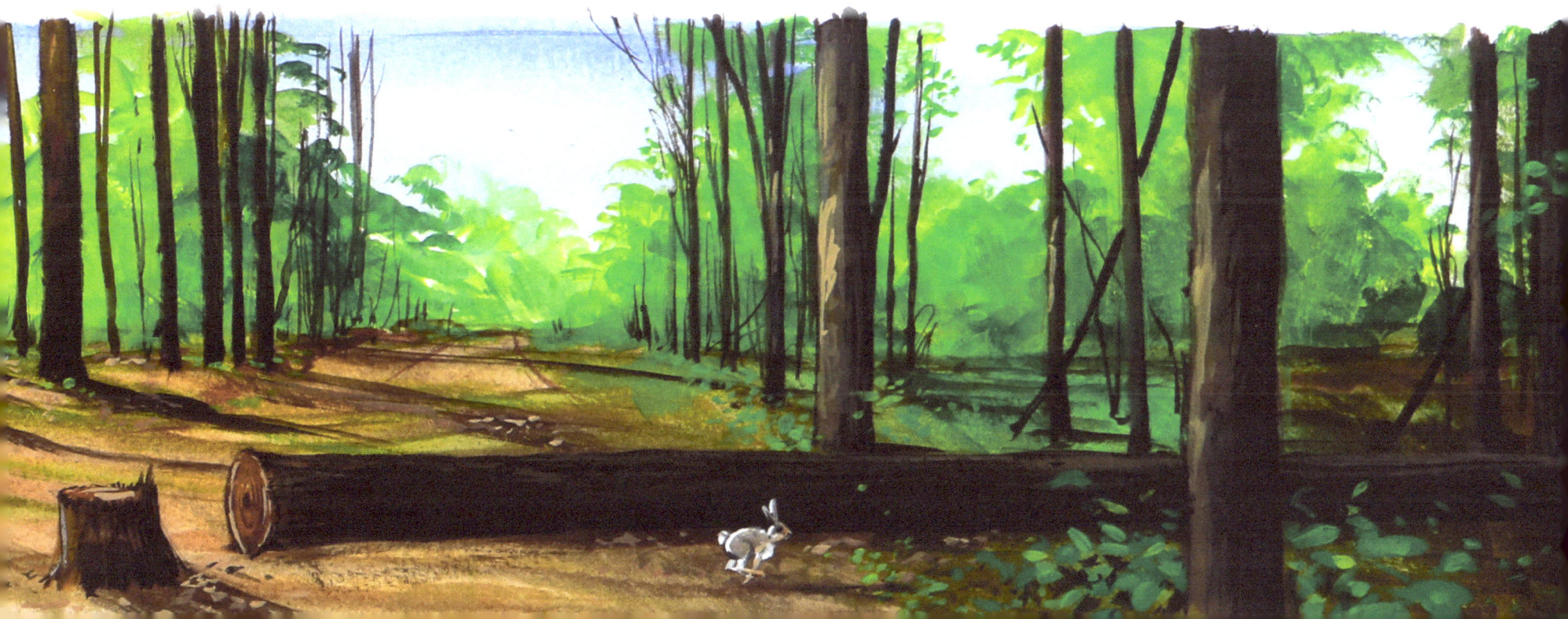

Fantastic once we know how to use it, but horrific if it's unbalanced, fabricating stuff which we accept as the truth, growing new horrible stuff on top of fabrications by increasing the intensity. All of which we believe to be real. That's a living hell which our Thinking Part (Arrogantio) has managed to create by insisting on bringing forward old 'spent emotions' that should have been managed, DROPPED and archived ages back. Mix that lot up with a good dose of FEAR and watch our system go into organism protection mode – all for no good reason without a shred of real danger in sight. Our bacterial side has no way to stop; it's designed to react to life with no way of telling what is real and what isn't real. An attack is an attack, until the point where the Thinking Part realises this is a false alarm. Our Thinking Part is the only part that can bring about change. Maturio must learn how to make changes without upsetting Habitu and Oucho or being sabotaged by Arrogantio.

Okay, so how do we manage so many changes without upsetting Habitu? Surely such a brilliant system would have a key to bring a quick resolution to this puzzle? And it does. That's where Maturio shines through as our hero bringing salvation. Maturio has a special ability to NOTICE glitches within our system and this is how it works:

- Maturio (in the Thinking Part) NOTICES glitches in the system;
- NOTICING the glitch alerts our body cells (in the Knowing Part) of the glitch;
- Our body cells alert our bacterial side (also in the Knowing Part);
- Once fully aware of the situation the Knowing Part auto corrects the glitch.

Maturio's only part is to NOTICE then keep out of the way while the Knowing Part corrects the situation. That's where so many of us fail because we find it too hard to keep out of the way. We fail to place trust in our own system and worry the job won't be done. Or simply fail to discipline our self to 'mind our own business'. When Maturio steps across the line into the Knowing Part's domain, more alarms are accidentally set off, kickstarting the old cycle all over again. Oops! Never mind, our early forgiveness prevents us from slipping into a punitive response and gets us out of the negative cycle. However, so many of us are unable to forgive and let go which is another blocker needing removal.

Maturio's ability to NOTICE doesn't come in glamorous packaging; it's quite bland and often discarded without activation. Like having a special piece of equipment that wouldn't work so we threw it away not realising it needed a

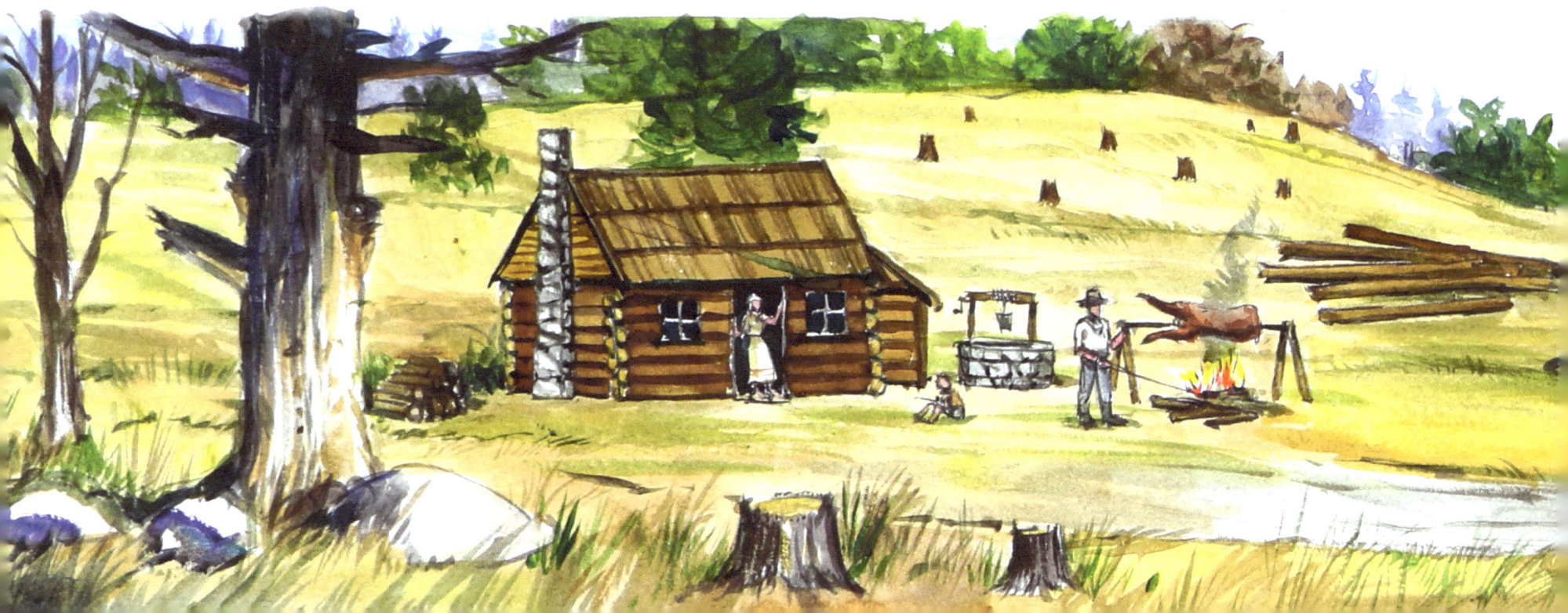

battery! However, when Maturio NOTICES Habitu's irrational habits the Knowing Part automatically hits the delete button. Phew! So that's how it's done! These changes are one hundred percent acceptable and activated without fuss or resistance. We might have realised such a brilliant system would have a built-in fail safe. Arrogantio has been trying to distract Maturio to prevent us finding the key. Maturio immediately forgives Arrogantio, knowing anger only gives more power to Arrogantio. At last, Maturio has learned it's more productive to suck it up, forgive and move on. That works – even if it does makes us want to vomit! We want the bigger picture of peace and tranquility and we will do whatever is necessary to reach our goal.

First Maturio needs to get free of Arrogantio to gain control which is difficult because Maturio starts off being quite weak and is easily derailed by Arrogantio. However, Maturio gains strength from learning to stand up to Arrogantio without becoming punitive, which would only flick Arrogantio to the fore and push our system into defense mode yet again. We make great progress once Maturio realises any form of self-destruction must be avoided. So that is our dilemma; how to gain control of one part without destroying or upsetting the other part. The answer is by clever negotiation and not by force.

Maturio must quickly learn two great skills:

1. How to respectfully negotiate with our giant bacterial side which looks after us by protecting our organism;

2. NOTICING.

At first Maturio makes plenty of mistakes before working out that anything that belongs to the Knowing Part must not be touched. Maturio must come to terms with the fact that it's not the boss of our symbiotic organisms and its area is only a tiny part of our organism; more like a pimple on a mountain. That's very painful for Maturio to accept, especially with Arrogantio putting up massive resistance and carrying on about being the omnipotent one. Maturio must find ways to forgive itself and Arrogantio for making these errors otherwise its own self-condemnation will trigger a negative response from our bacterial side. Exactly what we are trying to avoid. Once it has mastered all of that, before balance can be achieved Maturio must manage a variety of competing forces that are integrated and interconnected within us, all vying for power. Thankfully because our parts are interconnected, small changes correctly placed in one area can have a profound effect on other areas. This is the way that Maturio can make changes that are effective beyond its boundary. So, our success is all about

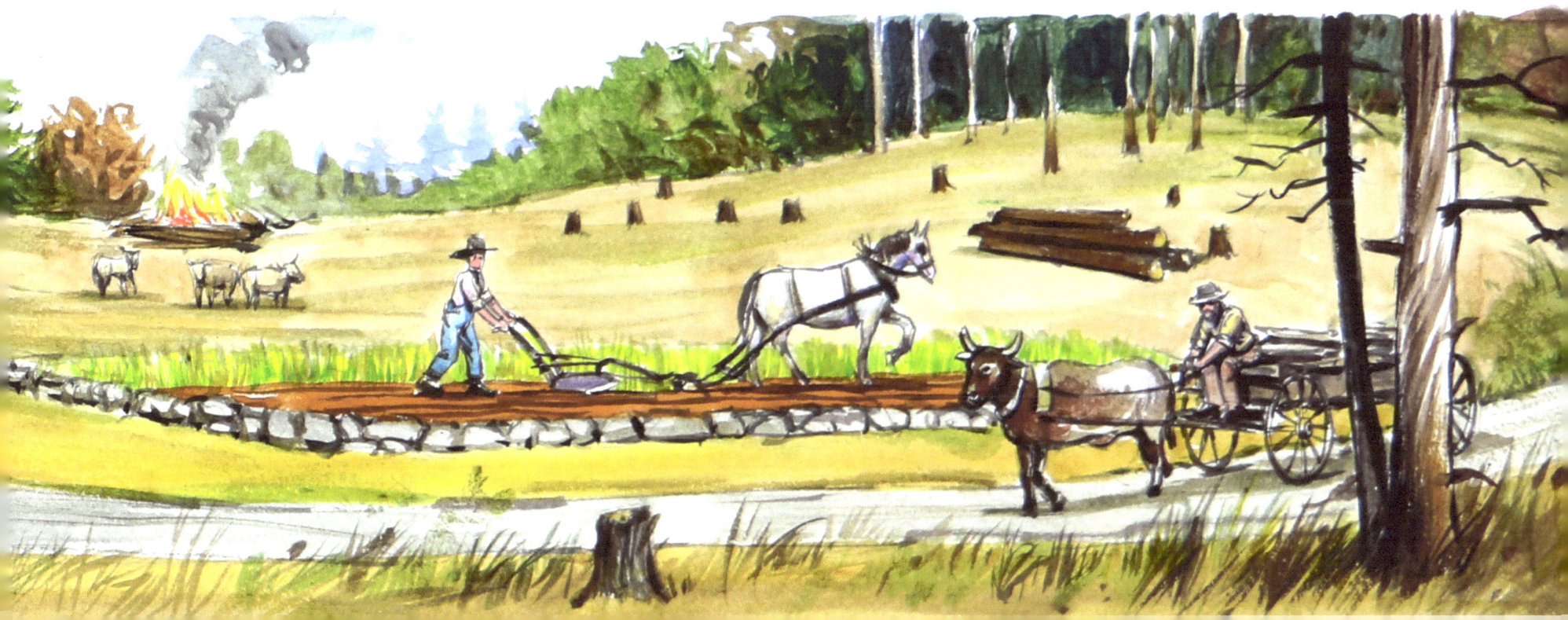

our Maturio learning to manage what can be managed and disciplining itself to leave the rest alone and because we are Maturio this is the dilemma we each face. Thankfully our task can be broken into manageable chunks and the chunks most in need of our attention are:

balancing LOVE and FEAR;

balancing Arrogantio and Maturio;

balancing Habitu's rational and irrational habits;

balancing fresh and memory feelings and emotions;

balancing how we use our Thinking Part and our Knowing Part.

Balance doesn't mean things have to be 50/50. For example, if we look at our selected chunks, a reasonable point of balance between LOVE and FEAR would be to have more LOVE than FEAR. How about 90% LOVE and 10% FEAR. For our Thinking and Knowing parts we might feel comfortable with 40% Thinking and 60% Knowing which puts the balance of power on the Knowing Part's side to remind the Thinking Part it isn't the boss yet gives the Thinking Part plenty of air space. For Habitu 90% rational habits and 10% irrational habits would be great but maybe too hard to achieve so let's aim for 75% rational and 25% irrational. For Maturio and Arrogantio how about 80% Maturio and 20% Arrogantio and the same would work for 'fresh' and 'memory' feelings and emotions.

We work out where the point of balance needs to be set, and we make adjustments so that our parts gradually become balanced. Wow, that's us taking responsibility for our own life! How exciting! Habitu will eventually form a beautiful new habit to keep us balanced and life becomes much easier. That's us working smarter using our special human gifts to their best advantage, turning stuff around to make the pre-historic system we inherited work for us and not against us because life gets ugly when our own parts work against us.

What will life look like if we start our journey with an unbalanced mess like this:

LOVE 10% FEAR 90%;

Maturio 10% and Arrogantio 90%;

Habitu running on 90% irrational habits;

Memory feelings and emotions 80% and fresh 20%;

Knowing 10% Thinking 90%.

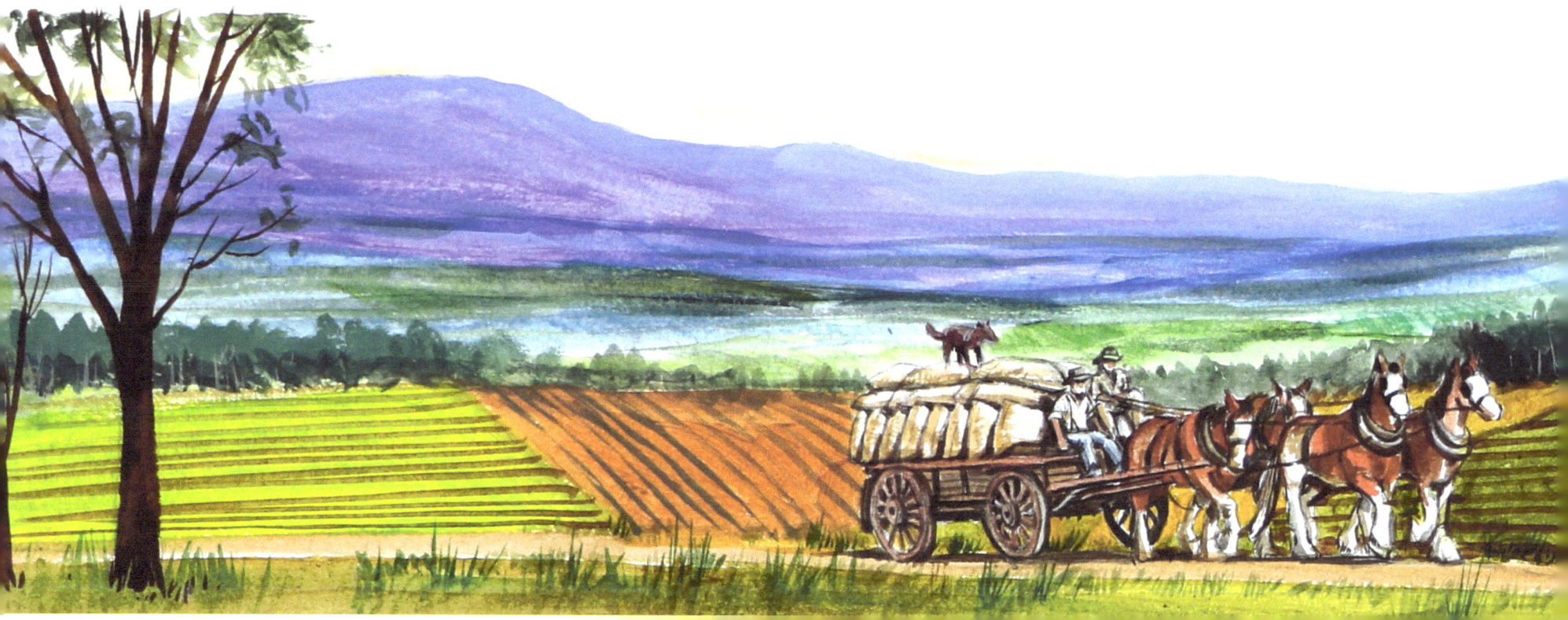

Okay that's a good insight into why life gets messy and provides a reasonable idea of where to make changes. Who would suspect simply changing the point of balance could have such a massive effect on our life? Obviously, it's going to be a confusing journey while Maturio discovers the parameters of such a complex web where touching one part alerts other parts; and only designated parts can resolve issues within certain areas. Get it wrong and trigger yet another repetitive false alarm to bounce uncontrollably between the Thinking and Knowing Parts creating living hell. At least we are working towards improving our choices.

By learning to NOTICE when our various parts are being manipulated, or even when we are trying to manipulate other people, we can slowly work out which of our thoughts, feelings and emotions belong to Alerto, Habitu, Oucho, Arrogantio and Maturio as these are the only clues we are given. Being able to SEE Arrogantio is a huge bonus but Arrogantio is the master of disguise, a chameleon and a shape changer so we are bound to make plenty of mistakes! As we gain a better understanding of when we are running on fresh incoming feelings and emotions and when we are running on memory feelings and emotions, we realise memory feelings and emotions can be used for positive or negative reasons; reflection and planning by Maturio or manipulation by Arrogantio and Habitu. We are learning to recognise the difference between them and becoming more selective. Previously our life was quite out of our control and we didn't even NOTICE – but we do now.

Slowing our mind helps us to SEE Arrogantio's control tactics because Arrogantio hates going slowly. We can listen to the bombardment of reasons to go faster. Good, we're learning to listen, soon we'll be able to SEE how this part uses 'memory emotions' to replace fresh new emotions to control us by preventing us experiencing new information coming in second by second. But is it Arrogantio or is it Habitu? Both will try to control us, and we need to know 'which is which' because each part must be addressed in a different way. Rushing could cause a nasty mistake which is another reason to slow down. The more we SEE the smarter we will be, however, Oucho will block us from SEEING anything painful – another blocker for Maturio to get around. And that is precisely what we are up against, block after block after block. Finding balance isn't easy but is achievable if we have oodles of patience. We are already relating differently; life is improving, and our new awareness is helping us to dodge some old mistakes.

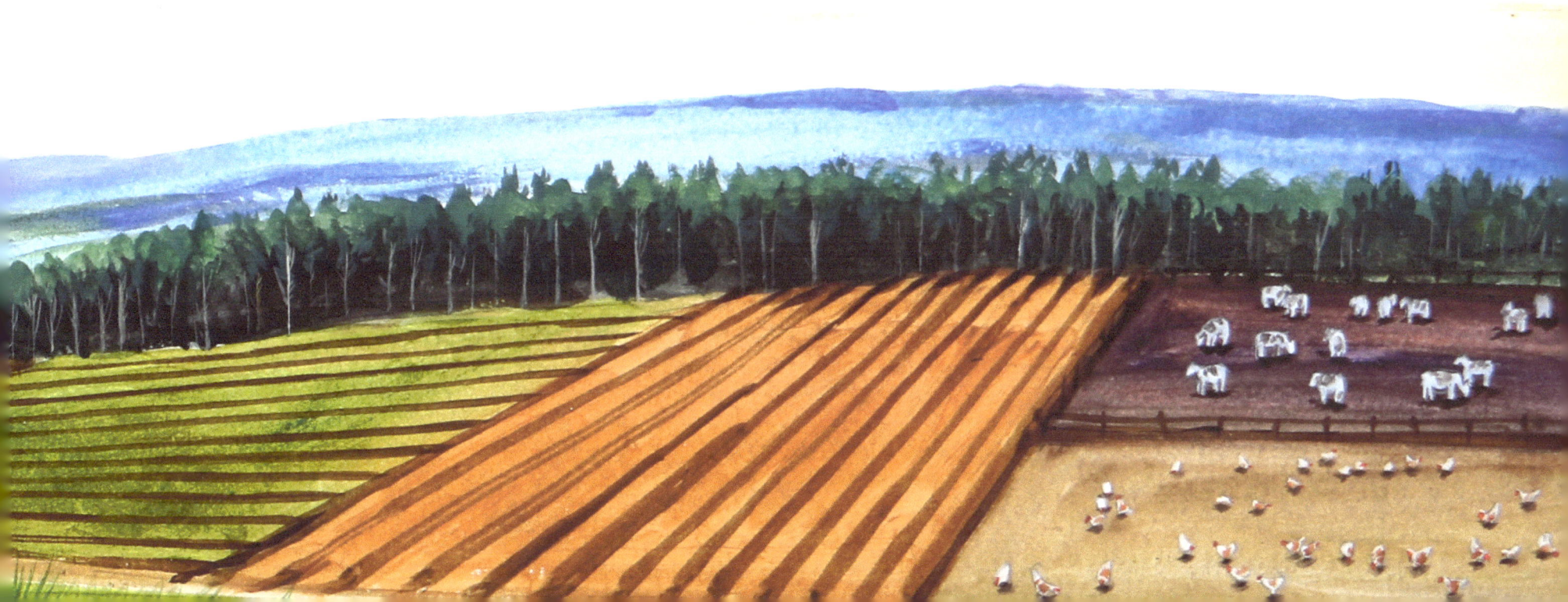

Something we do need to be aware of is that each of our organisms has a different focus on life. Bacteria 'live on' after our body dies therefore aren't as focused on staying healthy to live longer as the body cells are. Our bacterial side don't give a hoot about being balanced as they hardly know the Thinking Part exists. It's our Thinking Part that need to make all the effort and must be prepared to do whatever it takes to align the competing forces to become balanced because this increases our chances of longevity. If that includes dropping a bit of old garbage and putting fresh habits in place to stay alive longer, then that's exactly what we need to do. All our changes will be met with resistance which is part of the complex dance we need to perform to find balance.

Let's work to balance the chunk for LOVE and FEAR to give us an example of how the process unfolds; it doesn't matter where we start because our parts are integrated, change one, change the others. Right up front we know not to mess with real FEAR or real LOVE as both belong to our Knowing Part but we can work at reducing fabricated FEAR and increasing fabricated LOVE as both belong to our Thinking Part. We increase fabricated LOVE to create a place for LOVE until the real thing turns up, like putting a space aside in readiness. This

helps us to train Habitu to accept LOVE otherwise when LOVE does arrive Habitu will block it out.

If the LOVE within us feels like a hard shrivelled up pea, or has no feelings at all, it's time to fake LOVE to establish a position in our life for LOVE. We need to take care that we do not use this to replace LOVE because that doesn't work. We do it purposefully knowing it isn't the real deal. Just as our imagination can create false FEAR on top of real FEAR we're using the same process in reverse by creating a sense of false LOVE with a hope to one day the real LOVE will arrive. We are doing all that we can to mend our connection to LOVE.

To reduce FEAR, first we gather courage until we are ready. For some people confronting FEAR means facing up to scary childhood memories while others might be confronting horrifying hallucinations and monsters created by the mind. Or that wonderful wave of pure FEAR which floods in uncontrollably from nowhere to carry us off in its churning current. A useful strategy is to gain a tiny bit of control by confronting FEAR for just three seconds which is enough to start a change process. What a relief! To go to the next level purposefully increase FEAR's intensity for 3 seconds – one, two, three and back down. Just

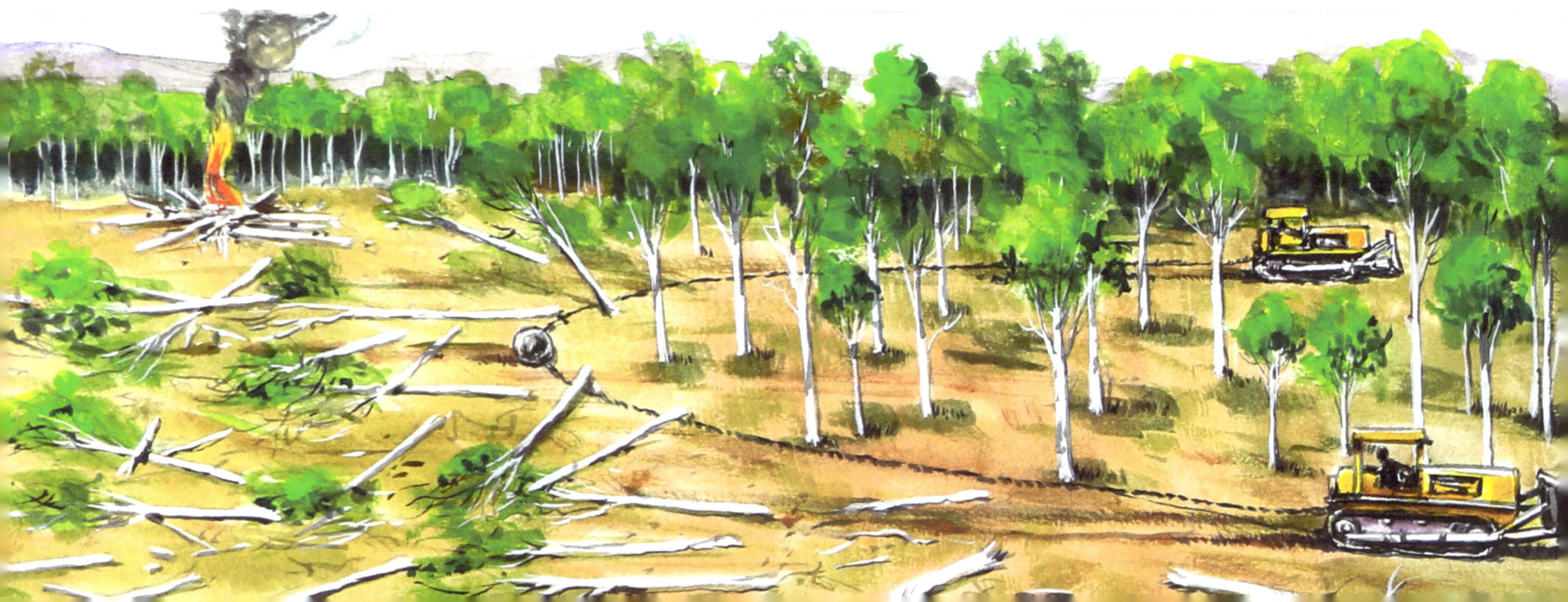

enough to let FEAR know the 'rules' have changed. When we are ready, move forward by doubling three seconds to six seconds, then twelve, then twenty-four and so on, growing stronger by the day. Standing firm for three seconds still may take months of preparation because we know there'll be a backlash, however we are ready.

As we watch 'FEAR' unfolding, we SEE that it's 'just a performance' with a regular routine which repeats itself over and over again. Part of us feels foolish and a little sick in the stomach while another part feels safer. We relax a little and suddenly we are blocked again! At first, we panic, like losing connection to our favourite TV show just at the crucial point. After a bit of pondering we realise Oucho has kicked in to protect us from the painful truth; but we are hungry to SEE, even if it is ugly. Maturio takes a humble approach to Oucho, respectfully approaching our inner giant and acutely aware that one tiny bit of arrogance will lock us out. Our success depends on Maturio's ability to control Arrogantio. We naively approach Oucho quite unaware of the backlog of painful unfinished business waiting to flood forward in one almighty whoosh. Oh no! Years of stuff parked around the body patiently waiting for a resolution. No

wonder millions choose to stay uncomfortably stuck and no wonder Oucho tries to protect us from experiencing this avalanche of pain.

We get it right: Oucho 'lifts a veil' and we SEE clearly. It overwhelms us; way too much and way too painful. At first, we are taken aback but realise our brilliant system allows us to park stuff for another time. We sense through messages coming in from our gut that this stuff is our GOLD. None of it belongs to today so it's safe to use to practice our newly developing communication skills. Honing our craft, getting our actions right for future events. However, our focus is managing FEAR and we don't need a distraction – which could even be Habitu or Arrogantio taking us OFF TRACK. So, we 'park' our golden garbage for another day. It's already been parked for years so a bit little longer won't hurt. Amazingly Oucho is happy because we are managing our pain and using our parts wisely. We sense the difference within. Having this small amount of control over our self feels good.

We return our mind to addressing FEAR and NOTICE how powerfully FEAR opens the performance, then something else happens. We SEE our imagination kicking in to escalate FEAR, triggering FEAR on top of FEAR, escalating to

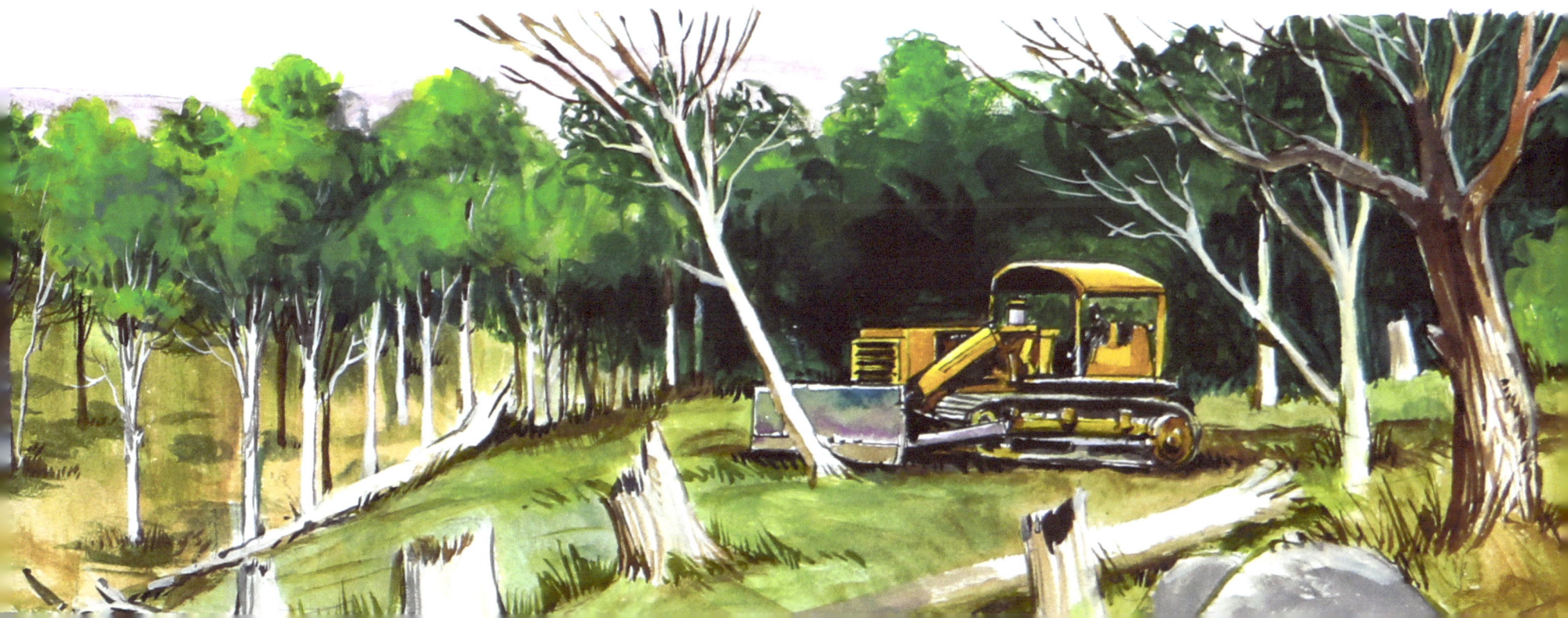

terror. We SEE the first part belongs to Alerto (Knowing Part) and the second part belongs to Arrogantio (Thinking Part). What a monumental breakthrough this is! We know NOT to touch Alerto but we can do something about Arrogantio. Yes! Definitely a breakthrough. We SEE that Alerto had responded appropriately to a perceived danger, but it was our Thinking Part that escalated FEAR to ridiculous heights leaving us feeling powerless for such a long time.

Ouch! A deep wound to our pride, like a spear piercing slowly through our body. We feel very foolish and angry to have unknowingly done this to our self. We cannot afford to slip into 'self-punishment' or we'll lose face with Oucho and must bear our pain graciously. We understand now that our vindictive ability to self-destruct is why Oucho protects us from experiencing pain. We realise we can make choices in how we choose to respond to life.

We have a vision of responding differently but it's too late, Habitu automatically kicked in and we slipped into our old behaviour pattern. Oucho is very disappointed which alerts Maturio who knows the moment has passed but NOTICES and resolves to get it right next time. Maturio encourages us to be kind and forgive our self for making a mistake because our kindness keeps us

balanced, but we fail again, and again. We put 'getting it right' on our practice list for another day and return to our task of FEAR management.

Taking extreme care to avoid Alerto, we focus on reducing Arrogantio's part. This much we can do but something is blocking us. Maturio asks the Knowing Part for advice. The answer comes up that old resentments are blocking us from using LOVE and forgiveness. Arrogantio and Habitu both receive benefits from hanging on to resentment, grievances and garbage. This habit prevents our connection to LOVE. Okay that means we have more work to do balancing Maturio and Arrogantio. We dedicate some time and eventually find a way to DROP some garbage and forgive our self. It hurts and leaves us feeling a bit naked but to our amazement it works. Alerto calms down. Well of course, we've stopped attacking our self.

Life momentarily feels good and suddenly FEAR returns stronger than ever! What's going on? We were going so well. Ah yes, but also upsetting Habitu. Maturio immediately takes a humble approach to Habitu, respectfully approaching the giant within; knowing one tiny bit of arrogance will lock us out. Maturio reassures Habitu that all is well and negotiates for Habitu to accept our

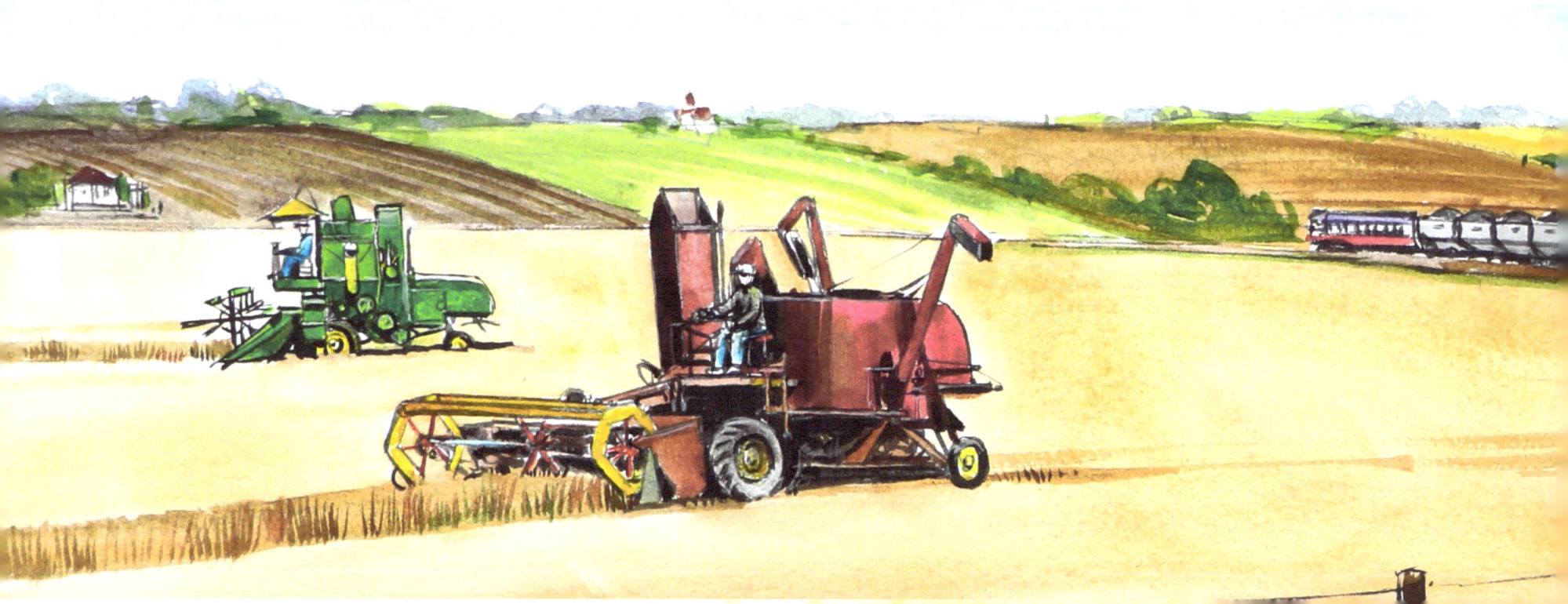

desired changes. Maturio is learning the importance of getting our timing right so listens carefully for our body's response before moving forward. If our gut hasn't settled, we talk to it with humility because it belongs to our Knowing Part. We ask is there anything wrong and reassure it that all is well. When our gut (Knowing Part) feels okay we move forward as a team, with all our parts working together.

One day we NOTICE that FEAR is no longer part of our day which feels rather strange. We humbly and respectfully ask Habitu to welcome 'strange' until these feelings become routine. Wow, we're getting our system to work for us and it's really happy to assist! Who'd have known we could do that! Life feels better with our parts pulling as a team. Naturally Habitu, Oucho and Arrogantio continue their sabotage, yes, but it's different now that we know their routine. We sit back, relax as the show unfolds and don't even take it personally. We SEE the clever control games; admire the ingenuity. Well done, nice try. We mostly manage to step around the games without getting caught and when we do get caught, we know it's better to acknowledge being tricked by a brilliant and masterful part of our self than falling into a sulk for being tricked. We're slowly

getting it right; our self-esteem is rising, we feel stronger and safer, listening to our gut more often and immediately know when a boundary has been crossed.

We understand the rules better now; LOVE and forgiveness get us off Arrogantio's hook; anger drops us deeper into the pit we're trying to escape from. We sense we are getting closer to reconnecting with LOVE, but something is in the way.

Another blocker! There must be some damage somewhere! We search for unloved feelings and find a small group we were ashamed of and tried to hide, but to feel fully loved we need to embrace all our feelings and emotions. Each has a special purpose, even though we don't understand what it is. For example, hate filled emotions are packed with angry energy; pocket rockets that can push us forward in tough times. Why waste this precious energy on childish angry outbursts when it could give us oomph to stick to our goals.

There are no bad parts of me –
but sometimes I use parts of me badly!

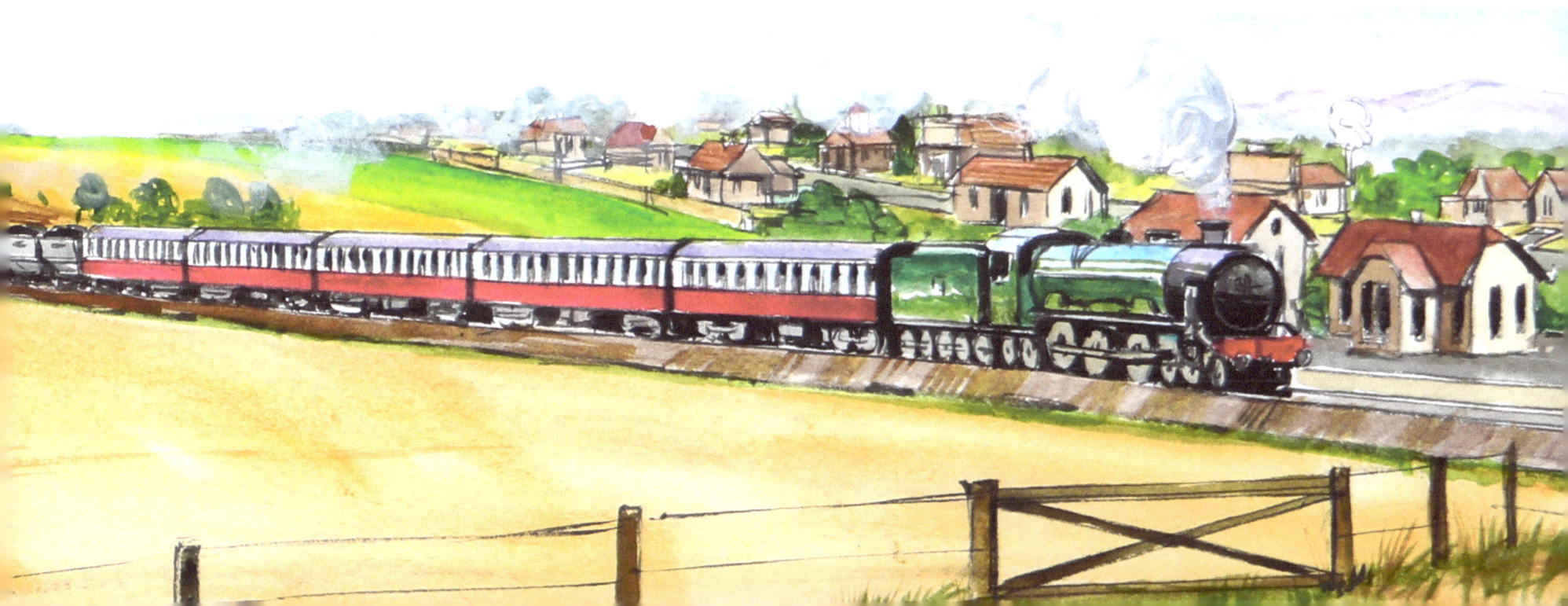

We trust the process and wait patiently while we guard our seeds of change from Habitu and Arrogantio who fill our head with negative self-talk and FEAR to back us off, but it's not so easy to put us OFF TRACK these days! We hold our hard-earned ground; conserve our energy for controlling Arrogantio. Wow, a functional new pattern is emerging. It feels good to know what we can control and what we must never try to control. Our timing is improving, life isn't such a mess and we feel our self stepping away from chaotic confusion, edging closer to a life of clarity and tranquility. That's different to how we would have responded a year ago, and that's how the process rolls forward.

Our defining breakthrough moment happens when Maturio finally realises that no matter what Arrogantio says, all of life's answers are not found in the head. Pressure is lifted as the Thinking Part stops fighting against the Knowing Part by placing trust in the gut. Maturio quickly realises both sources of information (memory and fresh) are needed to make sense of the world. Maturio SEES that although the Thinking Part plays a very important role, it's not the leading role 'it thought' it had to play which is a huge relief. Having worked so hard (in error) to 'best fit' information to guide the organism, Maturio now relaxes, happy to

be guided by the gut which brings in truth from the Knowing Part. Maturio still monitors the situation but now does so as part of a team.

That's balance!

It's time to introduce the last character from our bacterial side because once we are balanced we can harness this character's special powers to keep us on a steady track for the rest of our life. Aversio's creation was mentioned in Scene One where our forming symbiotic organism learned how to avoid eating poisonous plants, by putting down a deeply seated memory that would trigger future avoidance. Aversio uses deeply seated memory feelings and emotions to creates a powerful aversion. For example, if we overindulge in food to the point it makes us extremely sick – let's say chocolate cake – next time we glimpse or smell chocolate cake Aversio immediately triggers deeply seated memories which make us feel a little bit sick.

Cleverly done, because we hardly notice as we leave the chocolate cake and reach for something else to eat. Aversio is in the background guiding us all the time and can assist us to avoid repeating destructive or abusive behaviours that

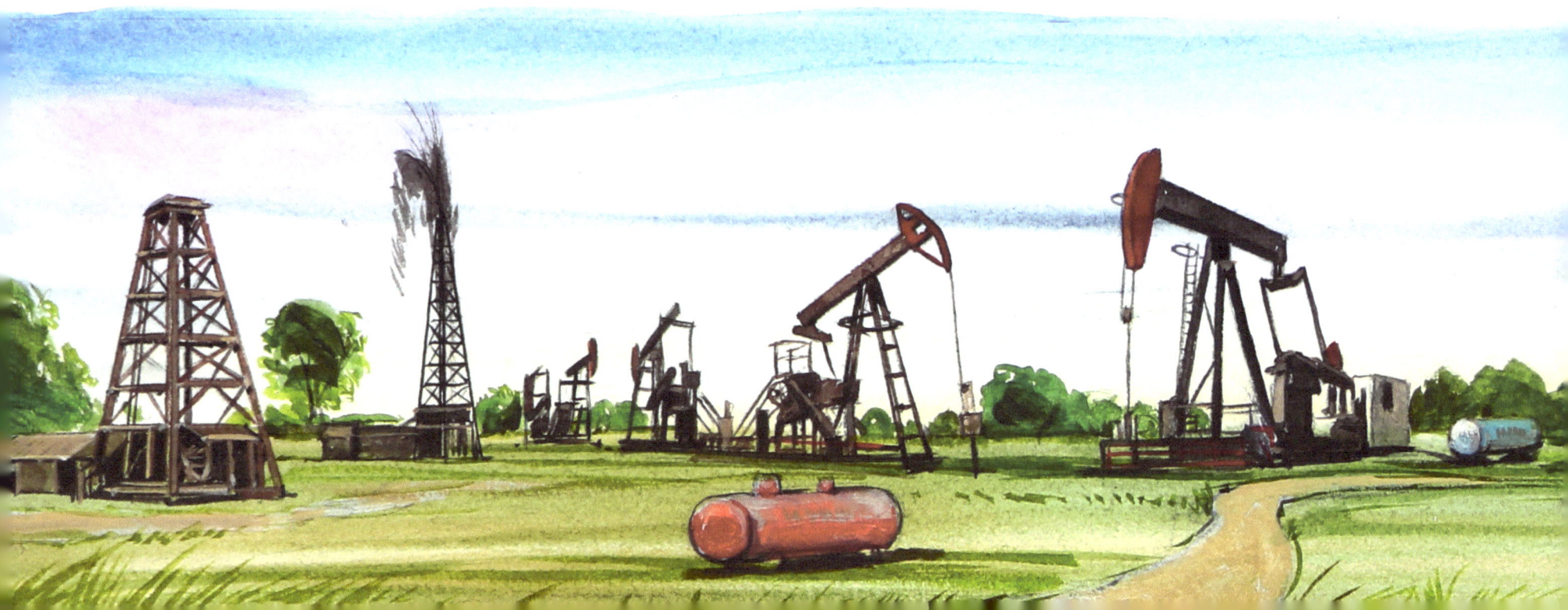

we would like to be rid of. First we must train Aversio by fully experiencing remorse to the point it makes us feel sick in the stomach; and at the same time we get very angry with our behaviour and make a strong resolve to never ever do that behaviour again.

Once these deeply seated memories are correctly in place Aversio will trigger each time we get close to breaking our own promise. Well, that's useful. No wonder our justice system always wants to know if a person is remorseful.

Are you able to identify the characters at work in these lives?

Please meet Fredrick

Fredrick's father was a mean man who beat his wife and children behind closed doors. Fredrick could never take friends home because his mother often had bruises all over her body. Fredrick learned to feign sickness on sports days, so his teachers wouldn't see the bruises on his body. He learned how to keep a low profile everywhere he went. When he grew up he didn't marry as he was afraid he would treat his wife the way his mother had been treated. He does his best to not let people see the rage that he knows is inside his body. He gets sick a lot and is on all sorts of prescription drugs; he's always at the doctors. People at the club like Fredrick but we don't really know much about him. He's going into hospital next week for bowel surgery.

Please meet Taliah

Taliah was very aggressive at school, and highly competitive. She would cheat her way through exams and had a knack of coming out of arguments that she caused looking like a saint. She's clever at manipulating people and appears to be a powerful leader. She gets a thrill from setting other people up to fail. I think she's quite dangerous to have around. Nothing bothers her, it's as if she doesn't have the same emotions as other people. I don't know why I keep her as a friend, she's done some terrible things to me. One time I ended up in court because of something that she did, and I took the wrap because all the evidence pointed in my direction. I felt so powerless, but she is so charismatic, and I remain fascinated by her.

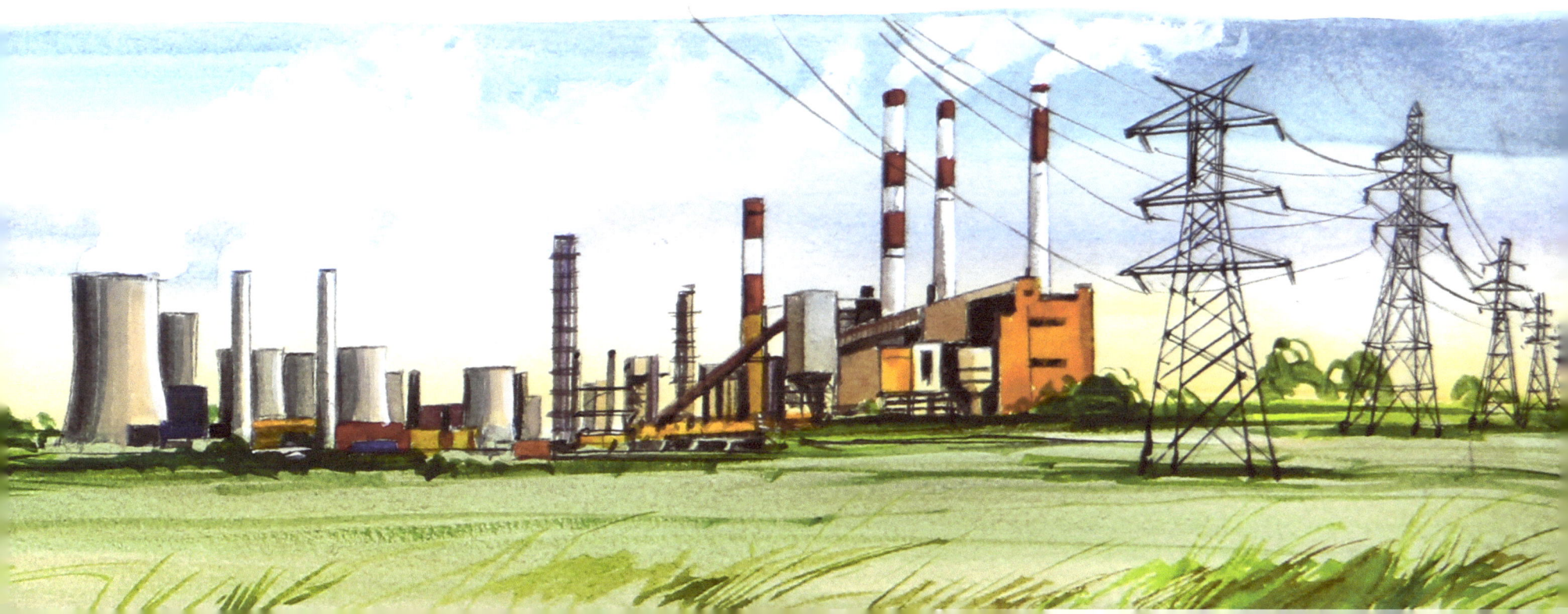

Please meet Catherine

Catherine is a fantastic person, always doing things for other people and has abundant energy which she invests brilliantly into her life. Catherine and her family have just as many hard times as other people, but she has a wonderful resilience to life and bounces back all the time. We are amazed at how much she gets done in a day. Her life is one big social whirl and her home is always filled with interesting people who resonate to her. She radiates health and wellness and looks years younger than her age.

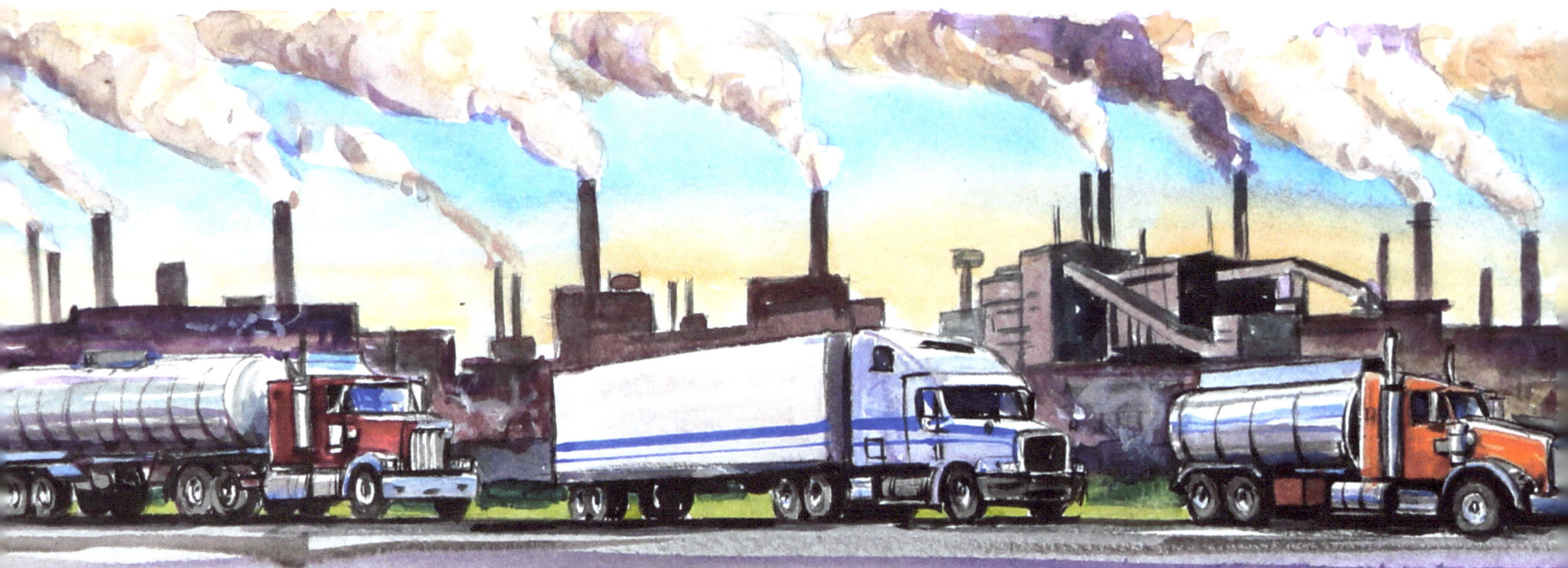

Scene Five – A New Day Dawning

It's difficult to comprehend how two tiny microscopic organisms managed to develop so much. A brain that could record information, control bodily functions, regulate body temperature, repair broken bones and flesh wounds, reproduce; and fill the body with LOVE for us to experience and share with each other. By design our body and mind are self-maintaining if we don't abuse them. Our happiness comes from fully accepting our self as we are, forgiving our self and others for errors of judgement, letting go of garbage and reducing false alarms.

Stuff happens to us all, no one knows when it's coming. Holding onto to old thoughts and memories doesn't protect us from new stuff coming in and although repetitive behaviours can give us a false sense of security it doesn't mean we're safe. Change is difficult as it involves stepping into the unknown which heightens existing FEAR which may already be paralysing the person. However, we shouldn't have a belly full of fear and racing mind unless we are about to be eaten by crocodiles which would perfectly explain this amount of stimulation. Unfortunately, millions of people needlessly live with screaming voices in the head and a belly churning with FEAR when there's not a drop of real danger in sight. Fully addicted to automatically responding to Arrogantio's scare mongering and Habitu's mindless need for predictable behaviours; sending millions of people reaching for the pills and potions. A chemical fix to calm the body and mind; providing a false sense of security and brief sense of relief. Life doesn't have to be this way.

Some people start their untangling process with nasty mental health illnesses that appear to be set in stone; some people are sickened by their own inability to control their behaviour feeling hopeless and helpless, while others hardly realise they have a problem. There are all sorts of reason why our life can get into a tangled mess. Thankfully once we demonstrate respect towards our bacterial side and manage to stand up to Arrogantio's bluff tactics, something deep within softens and the big scratchy old tiger melts into a sweet manageable pussycat. The crucial part is, will we be able to forgive our self for being trapped for so long; or will we reload shame, guilt, anger, resentment and hatred to return to the comfort of known behaviour. This is the true nature of the challenge we face.

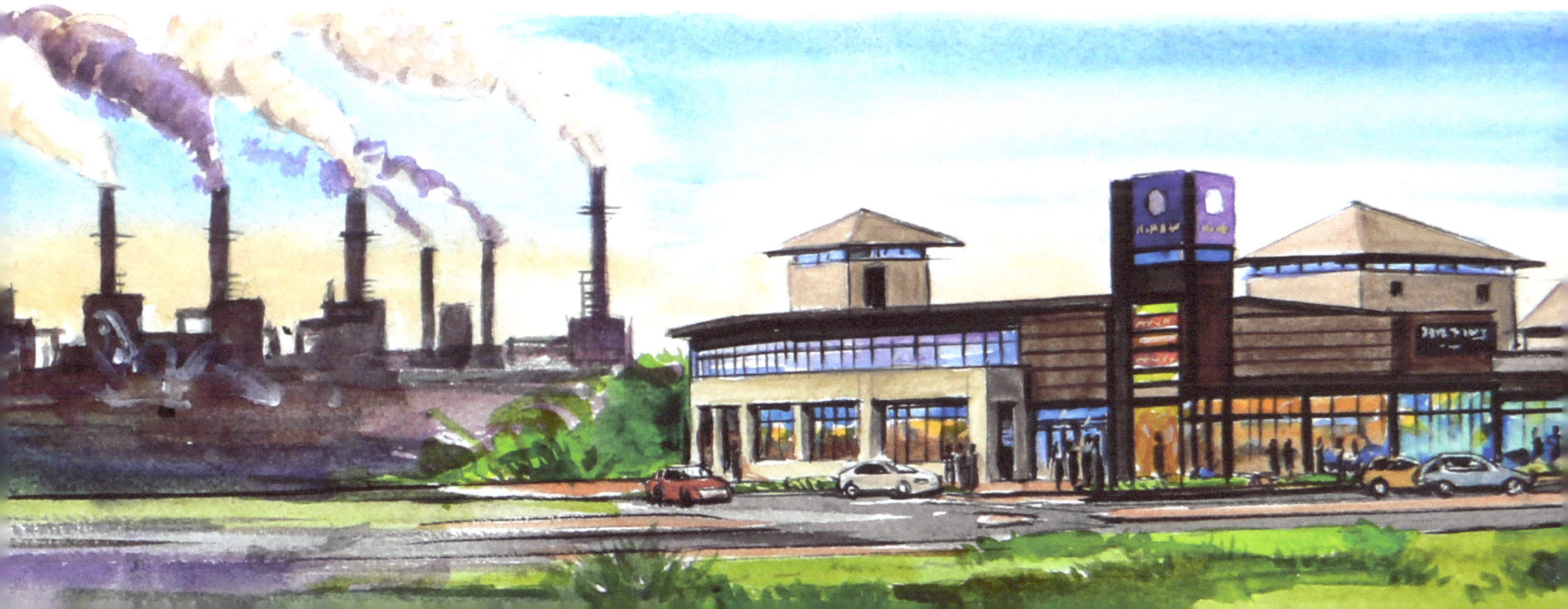

Forgiving and moving on is so powerful because it moves us to our LOVE side. We could almost say that Maturio is LOVE's child and Arrogantio is FEAR's child and that Maturio was lost when our connection to LOVE was lost. Finding Maturio brings us back to LOVE and takes us away from Arrogantio. If we find we cannot forgive, there's no need to panic as we can add 'inability to forgive' to our 'practice list' and spend quality time strengthening our resolve in preparation for the day when we decide to forgive. It's a big decision and involves dropping old resentments which Habitu has held in place, and besides that Arrogantio has told us we are justified to hold on to our resentment until we get a resolution, which Maturio knows will never arrive.

Every moment we spend re-living old pain is a moment lost experiencing today's sweet fresh life. Pain signals to our bacterial side that we are in danger. Oh dear, that's not so good! Next time the same old event is refreshed, it triggers an even stronger response. Why? Because our bacteria are trying to protect our symbiotic organism from an unknown regular attacker. When the attacker keeps returning they increase their efforts – which we experience as an escalation of FEAR. Keeping old pain 'refreshed' is very expensive, stressful to our body and a complete waste of energy. People who become 'stuck' in resentment for too long can become mean spirited. Some mean spirited people, blinded by Oucho, even hurt their own children and loved ones.

Human beings have the power to stop this behaviour by forgiving them self and others, dropping old resentments and emotionally moving on to a fresh new day. It's not a big deal, it's a little bit of discipline, a little bit of courage and the gradual formation of a new habit. Becoming 'stuck' in our thinking profoundly effects how we SEE the events of our day. If we look through eyes that only SEE garbage, we manifest garbage. This does not belong to LOVE, yet we do the manifesting. Time to wise up. Time for Maturio to start NOTICING as NOTICING gradually move us in the right direction; it links us to our gut which wants us to reconnect with LOVE. Be brave, trust our system, it will guide us to find balance. No need to panic, relax and trust that all will be well, in good time and eventually; and tell that little voice in the head (Arrogantio) to ping off.

NOTICING links our Thinking Part to our bacterial giant which is always happy to assist if we are wise enough to communicate in the language it understands, and that is LOVE. It's a simple recipe, LOVE opens communication and FEAR closes communication while the fight or flight response is activated. Where it all

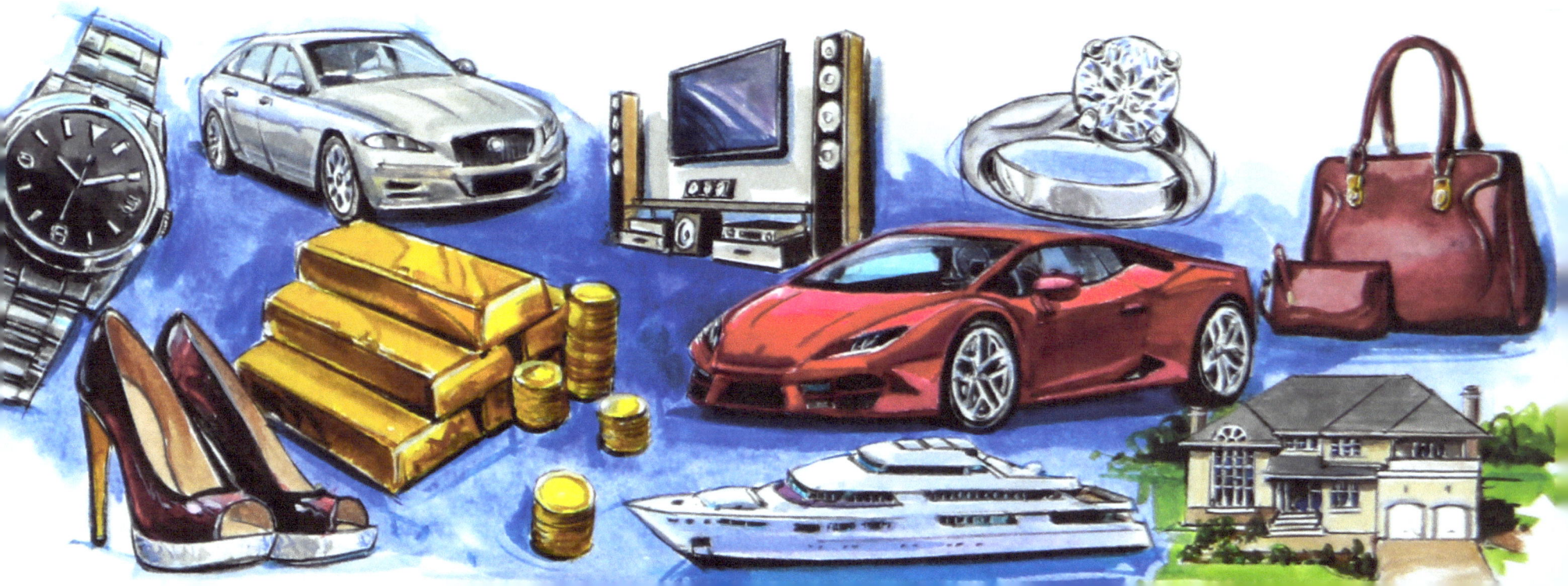

went terribly wrong is that our original design created a store of memories that could be quickly accessed to activate a survival response. However, language filled the same space with words. So instead of simply activating survival and moving back to LOVE, we got stuck in the Thinking Part – milling around in a sea of words, vulnerable to Arrogantio's desire for power.

Over many decades human beings allowed Arrogantio to bluff them into believing it was the boss; the all-knowing one, holding us longer and longer in the Thinking Part. We abdicated our power in exchange for a quick sense of safety; scammed by our own system. Although our mind is happy to accept this as the truth, our gut is not happy because it knows this safety is an illusion. It tries to alert us to look for the truth. Listening to our gut would prevent a whole lot of false alarms whereas ignoring it escalates the situation. Our task when a false alarm has been set off is to manage Arrogantio and bring Matuiro quickly to the fore so that we can return to LOVE. This is not the love we find in romantic novels or the love we might use to lure others into sexual encounters. This LOVE glues and binds our two organisms together; it's their communication channel where they share infinite knowledge with each other. Our bacterial giant is happy to work with Maturio to repair our connection to LOVE, we just

need to learn how to frame our requests in its language otherwise it cannot hear us. Sadly, sometimes our clumsy attempts to communicate do trigger false alarms.

Education systems and religions go on and on about the need to LOVE and forgive one another and so many of us thought that was about being kind to each other when really, it's so much bigger. LOVE is the pathway to connection with our full self, it opens portals to immense wisdom and knowledge, even vast information stored in our DNA. LOVE provides us with a deep connection to the universe and forgiveness gets us off Arrogantio's hook. We weren't so smart allowing Arrogantio to prevent us from living in the moment – killing that flicker of nervousness – that keeps us in touch with life. We can trust that 'slightly nervous' sensation to look after us because it's that 'slightly nervous' sensation that guides us all of the time. We need to learn its language and wake up to Arrogantio's trickery.

Knowledge in the Knowing Part is alive and fresh, and it refreshes us; knowledge in the Thinking Part is a recording from our past and has no life connection. No matter how cleverly crafted by Arrogantio, it can never replace information

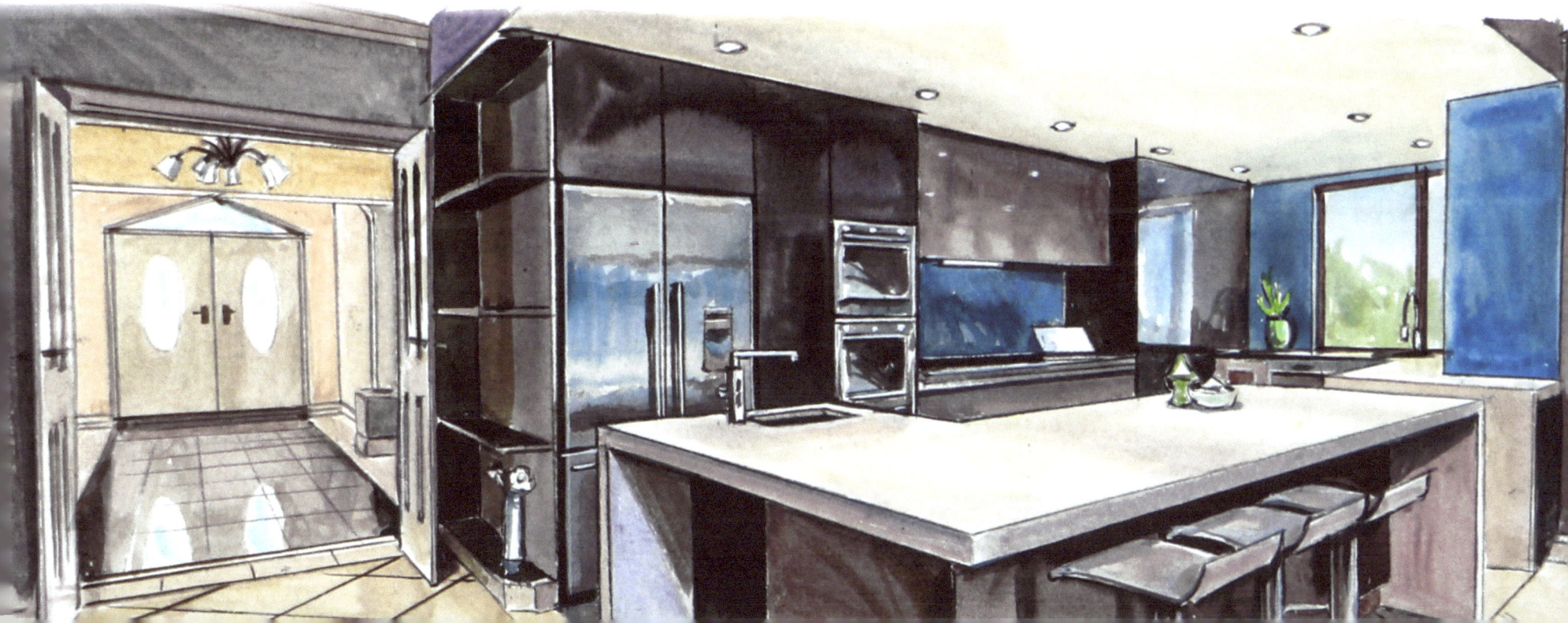

from the here and now. It's 'stale mail' not fresh mail. Habitu causes us to place too much trust in stale mail because it's 'known' and feels safer than fresh mail. However, stale mail leaves us running on semi factual information which cannot possibly keep us safe. We all struggle with the same dilemma of being able to get past Oucho to SEE what's going on so that we can manage Arrogantio and bounce back to LOVE which is our natural state of being. Humanity is so overdue to gain greater understanding of how our symbiotic organism functions. We need to learn to keep Maturio to the fore so that we can communicate with Alerto, Habitu, Oucho and Aversio from our loving side, because our punitive side only serves to trigger Alerto into fight or flight and places us under the control of Arrogantio. Simple mathematics. We are either experiencing LOVE or FEAR. FEAR activates our survival mechanisms and LOVE activates communication between all our cells and links us to the outside world. Living in the moment does take a bit of getting used to as it comes with a sense of uncertainty of what is coming next; Arrogantio and Habitu hate not knowing. We can't do anything about Habitu but we need to be ready and willing to forgive our self for getting things wrong because we will be repeatedly tricked by Arrogantio. Instead of wasting precious time worrying about falling into Arrogantio's traps, it's better to assume we will be tricked so that we can be

at the ready with our most powerful antidote – forgiveness. Maybe we didn't understand how to use it, but we have a much better idea now.

Maybe it's time for us to think about what life is like from our bacterial side, sharing a body with parts that trigger false alarms and create FEAR in the absence of danger. Luckily, our symbiotic organism functions independently to our Thinking Part which still only exists within the small subsection put aside for the body cells to create language. Our Thinking Part is ignorant of the incredible ability and knowledge held by the rest of the brain and body, only gaining glimpses when fully balanced with the Knowing Part. There is an incredible world of knowledge for us to explore once we get our self balanced, with Maturio to the fore.

This story has provided insights into what gets in the way of our connection to the LOVE energy within us, which has the power to connect us to all living matter. It radiates a sense of safety and wellbeing to everything it encounters. It communicates without words directly from the body because words cannot encompass the vast knowledge carried by LOVE energy which links and joins everything together. The next story can be written by you. A wonderful story

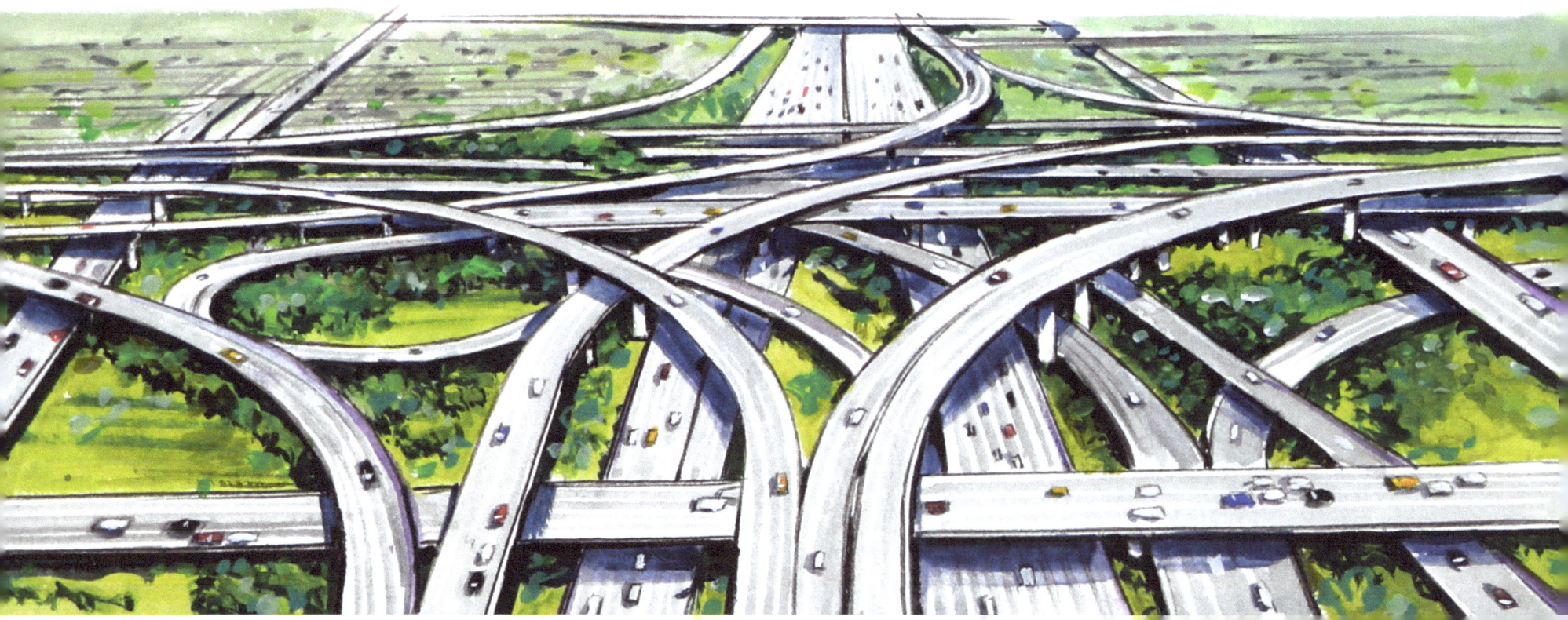

of how you found your way back to the LOVE within. That story will be about how you took up the challenge, walked boldly forward knowing all about Alerto, Habitu, Oucho and Aversio, the bacterial characters interacting within you, holding you to predictable pathways and constantly getting you OFF TRACK of your goals to change.

That story will tell of trials and tribulations as you worked your way through the maze – gathering insight and wisdom, realising how often you have unknowingly triggered false alarms to flood your system with FEAR. Learning to recognise Arrogantio's tricks; being filled with healthy pride each time you manage to step over and around the traps; understanding the bigger picture in your life and responding with forgiveness and LOVE instead of aggression and hatred. Doing the best you can to live peacefully in a world that can easily become chaotic. Doing your bit to spread LOVE not FEAR into your day. Learning to feel safer in your own skin by not fearing FEAR when it does come into your day. Putting something better into your DNA ready for the next generation to carry forward.

We live in an era that is about to explode with Artificial Intelligence where robots and computers will take over our daily grind. Perhaps this era will provide the dawn of a time where people will have time to find balance by NOTICING how their parts interact, learning what parts to take charge of and what parts not to interfere with. Learning to make a connection to the abundant supply of LOVE that is within us all. Our lives would be balanced, our relationships would flourish, we wouldn't be afraid of making mistakes and being wrong, there wouldn't be any need to fight each other or have wars. Our children would feel safer and our lives would be productive and satisfying. We would lovingly look after each other, our young, our elderly, our disabled and our self.

Our new position doesn't come with bells and whistles blowing. It's more of a calm sense of being fully connected with a safe and powerful life force within, however our outlook changes dramatically. We no longer mindlessly attack our self and feel more secure within our own skin. In case you hadn't noticed this whole story has been about how FEAR is used to control us and how we eventually learn to manage FEAR and reduce false alarms. When we embrace our vulnerability, we become stronger through being free of the need to pretend we are strong. We have more energy at our disposal and our life can be open and honest. When we stop being afraid we start to hear those delicate messages coming from our gut.

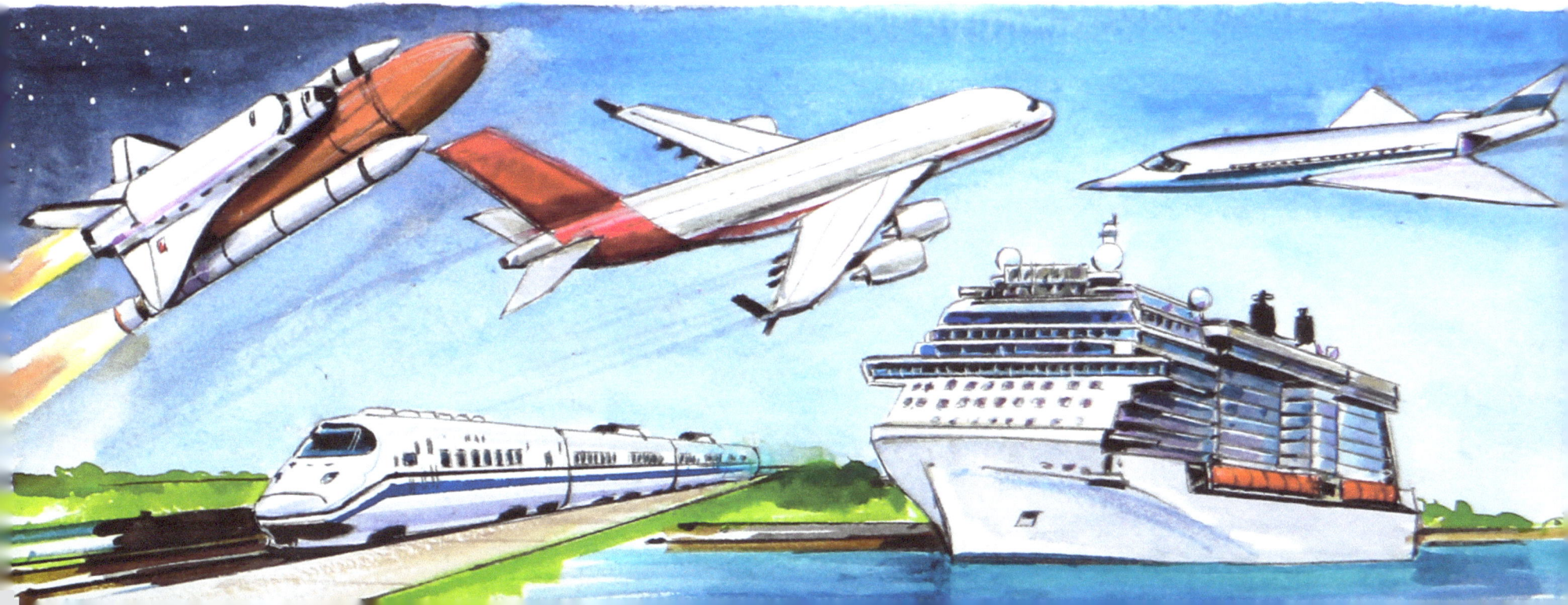

As we listen attentively, our entire system sighs in relief as we reconnect to LOVE. That's the turnaround we are looking for! This partnership was never going to happen while you and I selfishly hung on to our old rubbish, were too arrogant to forgive our self and others for mistakes, triggered false alarms and arrogantly thought we were the boss of the outfit. No way; and to make that perfectly clear, you and I are midgets working in partnership with a giant because we share our body with a massive colony of bacteria; they are the largest part of us. Our bacterial side is not the problem, Arrogantio in our Thinking Part is the problem. That's our most important part to work on until such time that we manage to find balance which will flood truth into our system. As truth releases into our Thinking Part, energy blockages are dissolved. Some people experience feelings and emotions which don't belong to them. It doesn't matter; relax, let it go so that everything is released and gone forever. We discipline our self not to become involved with these old emotions even if they scream for attention. We inherited a brilliant system with the capacity to receive a lot of telepathic information. Be vigilant and let it go! Some people might experience a temporary increase of faecal matter; physical evidence of the cost of hanging on to unresolved issues.

What an incredible system that given the right circumstances it can reorganise and fully cleanse itself. Who'd have known dropping a bit of emotional garbage and addressing a few toxic habits could be so powerful. Our face flushes with vitality as blood flow returns to maximum flow releasing sexual energy to pulse through our body. We glow with health and look attractive to others. Food tastes better, eye sight is clearer, hearing sharper, colours are brighter. We pick up so much more of what is going on around us; we're much more resilient and less likely to be manipulated. We feel reborn, refreshed and cleansed of garbage. We look through eyes of kindness, feel lighter and have abundant energy. Yes, it was a tough journey working with so many competing forces all vying for control, just getting past Oucho was so difficult but the results are amazing.

If all the people in the world were happy and fulfilled, I wonder if humans would be kinder to each other and to the planet we call home.

It's only a new habit away.

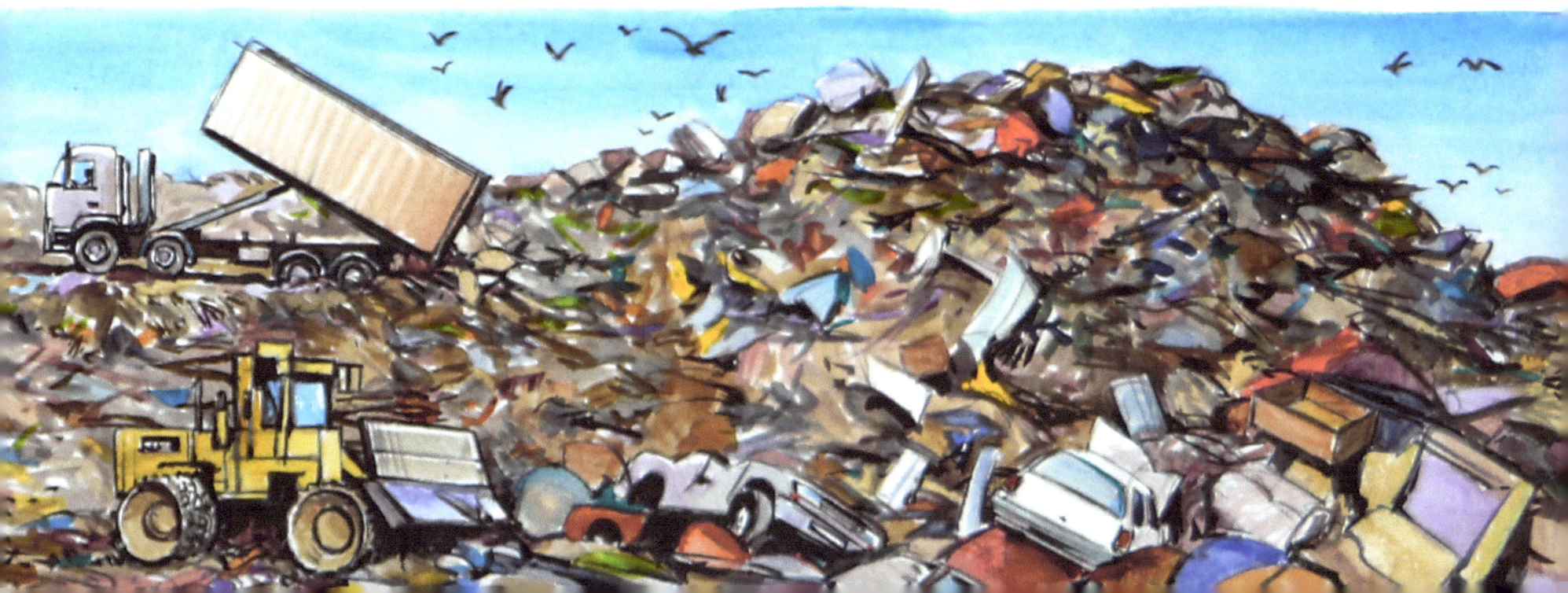

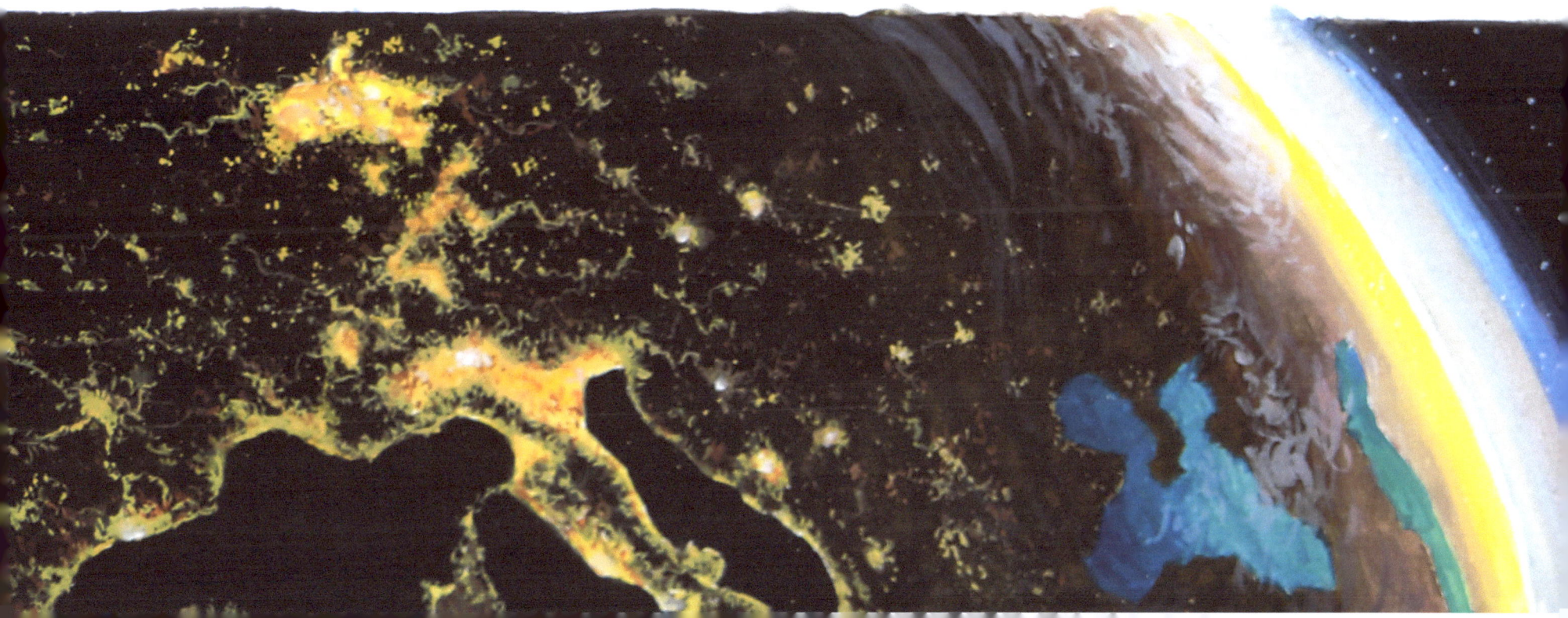

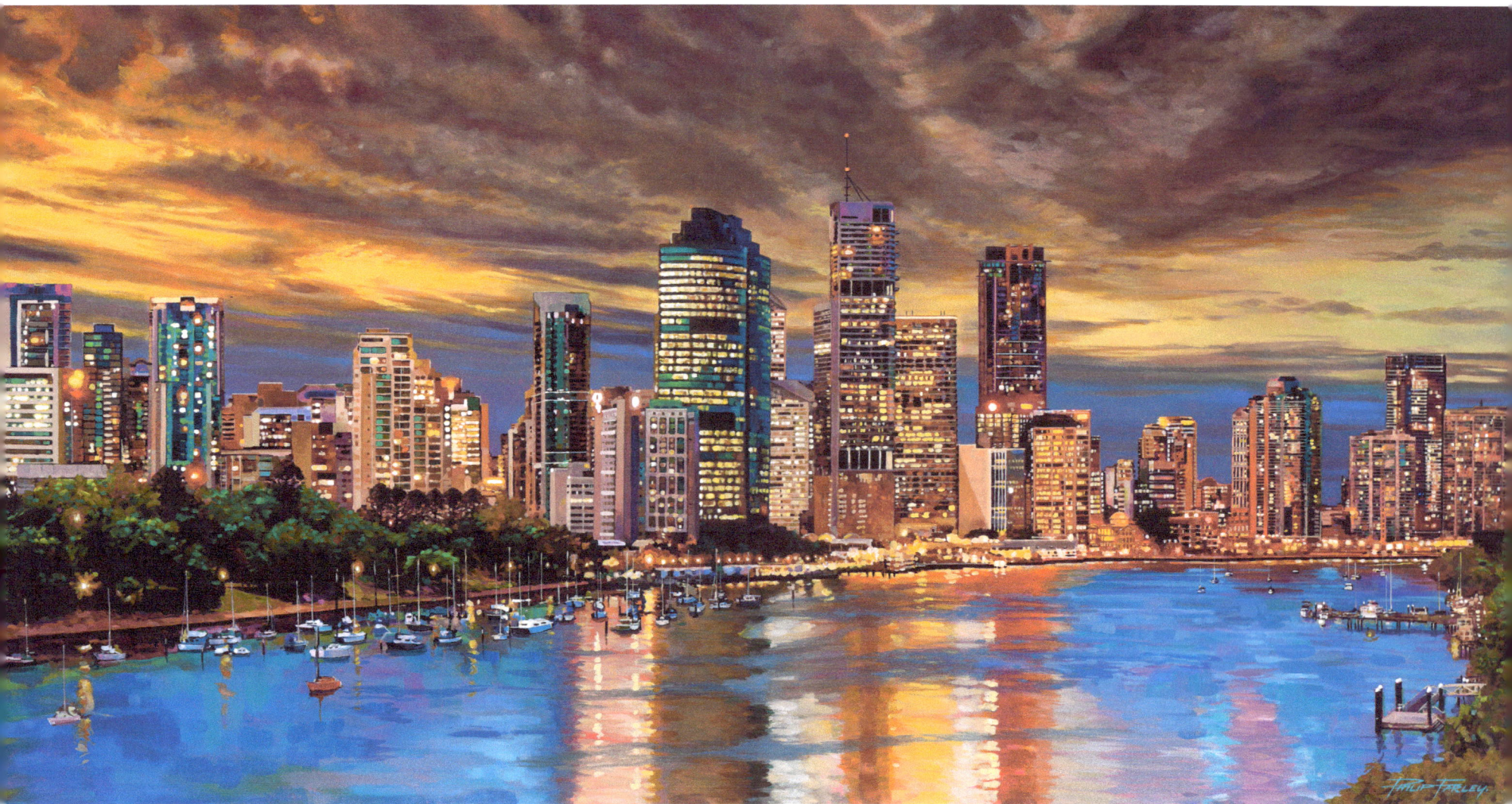

River City Glow

by Philip Farley

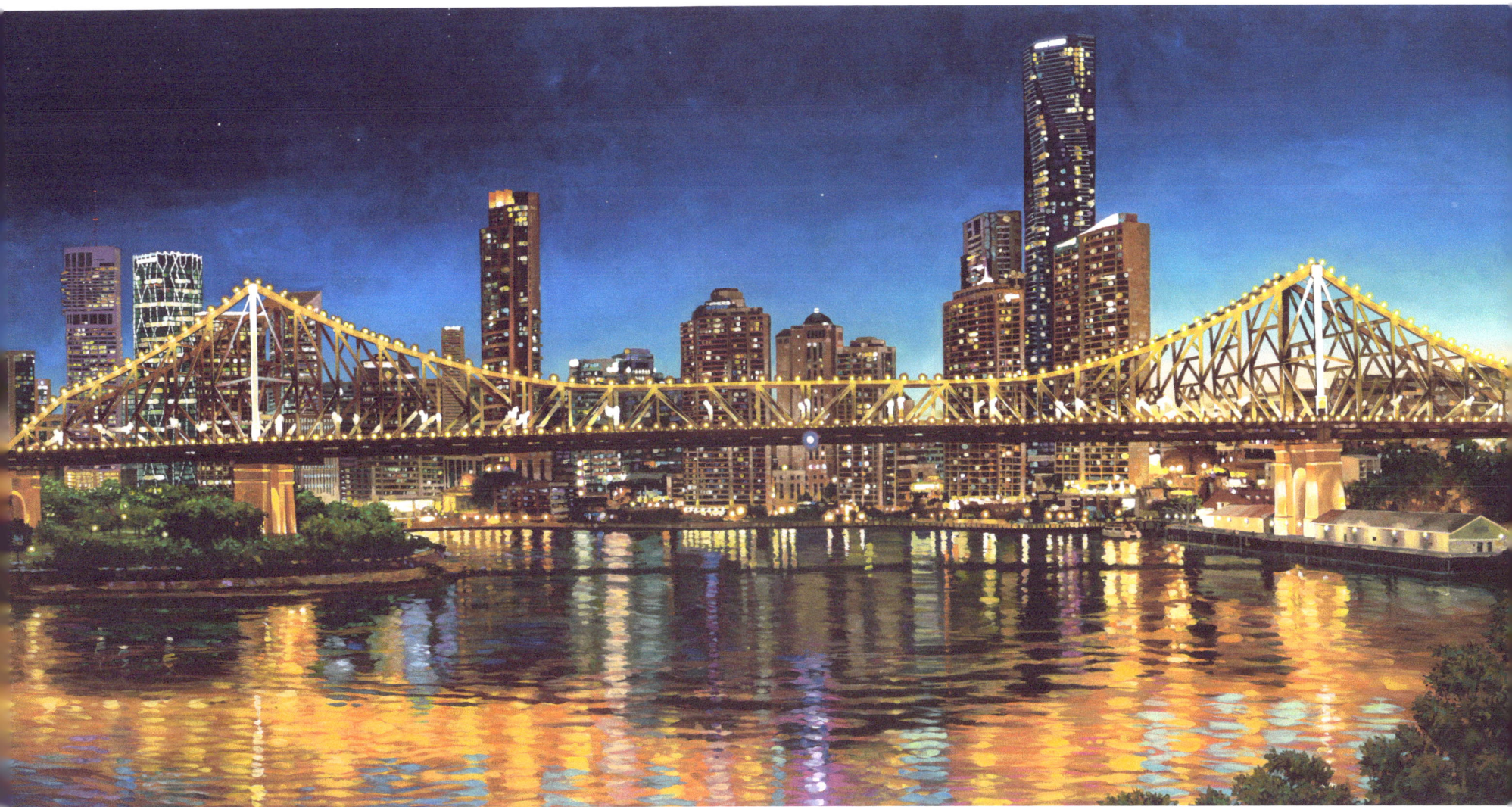

Bridge Reflections

by Philip Farley

It's your life
Get it sorted

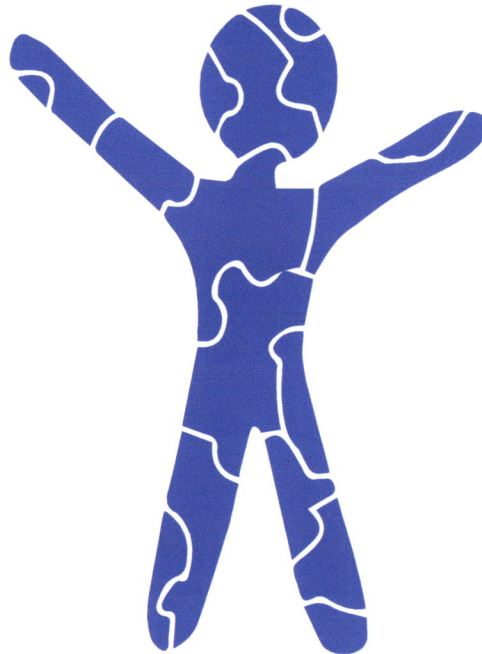

FragilePuzzle.com

Email: info@fragilepuzzle.com